THE ANATOMY AND PHYSIOLOGY OF SPORTS MASSAGE

Portia B. Resnick, PhD, ATC, BCTMB

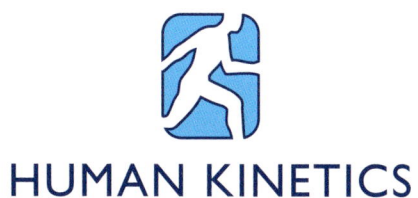

HUMAN KINETICS

Library of Congress Cataloging-in-Publication Data

Library of Congress Cataloging-in-Publication information is available.
LCCN 2025041628 (print).

ISBN: 978-1-7182-3821-3 (print)

Copyright © 2027 by Portia B. Resnick

Human Kinetics supports copyright. Copyright fuels scientific and artistic endeavor, encourages authors to create new works, and promotes free speech. Thank you for buying an authorized edition of this work and for complying with copyright laws by not reproducing, scanning, or distributing any part of it in any form without written permission from the publisher. You are supporting authors and allowing Human Kinetics to continue to publish works that increase the knowledge, enhance the performance, and improve the lives of people all over the world.

To report suspected copyright infringement of content published by Human Kinetics, contact us at **permissions@hkusa.com**. To request permission to legally reuse content published by Human Kinetics, please refer to the information at **https://US.HumanKinetics.com/pages/permissions-translations-faqs**.

This publication is written and published to provide accurate and authoritative information relevant to the subject matter presented. It is published and sold with the understanding that the author and publisher are not engaged in rendering legal, medical, or other professional services by reason of their authorship or publication of this work. If medical or other expert assistance is required, the services of a competent professional person should be sought.

The web addresses cited in this text were current as of August 2025, unless otherwise noted.

Senior Acquisitions Editor: Michelle Earle; **Developmental Editor:** Amy Stahl; **Copyeditor:** Christina West; **Proofreader:** Deborah A. Ring; **Indexer:** Kevin Campbell; **Permissions Manager:** Laurel Mitchell; **Senior Graphic Designer:** Sean Roosevelt; **Layout:** MPS Limited; **Cover Designer:** Keri Evans; **Cover Design Specialist:** Susan Rothermel Allen; **Photographs (cover and interior):** Kirk Fitzek/KF Studios; **Photo Production Specialist:** Amy M. Rose; **Photo Production Manager:** Jason Allen; **Senior Art Manager:** Kelly Hendren; **Illustrations:** © Human Kinetics; **Printer:** Versa Press

We thank California State University, Long Beach in Long Beach, California, for assistance in providing the location for the photo shoot for this book.

Human Kinetics books are available at special discounts for bulk purchase. Special editions or book excerpts can also be created to specification. For details, contact the Special Sales Manager at Human Kinetics.

Printed in the United States of America   10 9 8 7 6 5 4 3 2 1

The paper in this book is certified under a sustainable forestry program.

Human Kinetics
1607 N. Market Street
Champaign, IL 61820
USA

United States and International
Website: **US.HumanKinetics.com**
Email: info@hkusa.com
Phone: 1-800-747-4457

Human Kinetics' authorized representative for product safety in the EU is Mare Nostrum Group B.V., Mauritskade 21D, 1091 GC Amsterdam, The Netherlands.
Email: gpsr@mare-nostrum.co.uk

E9944

Contents

Foreword v ■ Acknowledgments vii

Introduction: Unraveling Some of the Mystery ix

PART I: Foundations

1	Muscles and Fascia	3
2	The Physiological Effects of Manual Therapies	17
3	Types of Manual Therapies	29
4	Structural Versus Functional Considerations	43
5	Common Compensations in Sport	63

PART II: Techniques

6	Shoulder, Arm, Forearm, and Hand	73
7	Upper Back and Neck	113
8	Lower Back and Abdomen	133
9	Hip, Thigh, and Knee	151
10	Lower Leg and Foot	181
11	Self-Care	201

Bibliography 215 ■ Index 217 ■ About the Author 229

Earn Continuing Education Credits/Units 230

Foreword

Manual therapists who work with athletes have to make clinical decisions on behalf of clients and patients who put unusual stresses and demands on their bodies. Competent practitioners need extensive knowledge of anatomy and physiology, but even more, they need to be able to apply these abstract concepts to the problems that their clients and patients face.

In *The Anatomy and Physiology of Sports Massage*, Dr. Resnick combines three critical domains of knowledge: her extensive understanding of how manual therapies affect function, her mastery of muscular and fascial anatomy, and her experience of working with athletes from a wide variety of sports. The result is this wonderful interdisciplinary resource. This guide is invaluable to massage therapists, physical therapists, athletic trainers, and many other practitioners, along with their patients. It is not easy to navigate the complex challenge of applying technical physiological concepts to the in-the-moment needs of athletes in training or recovery. This book bridges that gap between theoretical understanding and hands-on decision-making.

As a writer and educator who finds it all too easy to get lost in the minutiae of every topic, I especially appreciate Dr. Resnick's unerring focus on practical application of concepts. Every idea is presented with a "this is why you need to know this" explanation. This guide is far more than a textbook that will be left on a shelf after a course is completed. It is a lifelong resource and guide for safe and effective practice.

Ruth Werner, BCTMB (ret.), author of *A Massage Therapist's Guide to Pathology*

Acknowledgments

The human body is amazing and has fascinated me for decades. As a student and teacher, I have studied the body, but being a clinician and being able to put my hands on the body has taught me so much more. For that reason, I want to start by thanking every athlete, patient, and client who has let me work with their body. Thank you to my anatomy instructors for always challenging me, and thank you to every student who has put up with my nerdiness in class.

Special thanks to James (2012-2013) and Sarah (2014-2015), who donated their physical bodies to the Willed Body Program at the John A. Burns School of Medicine in Honolulu, Hawaii. You were both my greatest anatomy teachers, and I cannot thank you and your families enough for your selflessness. Mortui vivos docent.

Thank you to my family. E mālama i nā kupuna.

Everyone should have a team like mine who is there to support them. In no particular order, thank you to my sister from another mister and the husband (Audra and Mike), my trifecta (with Ali and Abbi), quartet (with Karyn), antagonists (Kathy and Kristen), office mate (Kara), and gnomies (Reggie and Mike). Special thanks to Big Ben, the dog, for reminding me I am never too busy to take a walk or play hallway tennis ball, and his human, Michael, for encouraging me to get out of my comfort zone by doing something that scares the heck out of me.

Finally, thank you to everyone at Human Kinetics for giving me this opportunity, especially Michelle Earle. It wasn't the project you originally posed to me, so thank you for letting this become my vision.

Introduction: Unraveling Some of the Mystery

The Anatomy and Physiology of Sports Massage is designed to support practitioners who use manual therapy as part of clinical practice, providing guidance on the types of manual therapies, their role in exercise recovery, and their use in treating and preventing chronic musculoskeletal injuries. Combining the understanding of the physiology and the intent behind different manual therapy techniques with the anatomy helps ensure the correct outcome, allowing a variety of clinicians to understand the role of the muscles and how to create effective manual therapy treatments. Manual therapy instructors can use this book as a reference on the why and what of sports massage, going beyond just techniques. For students, this comprehensive guide provides answers to many questions in one place.

Many types of health care professionals use manual therapy in their practice to work with athletes and other active individuals. Although massage therapists may be proficient in their manual therapy skills and in the physiology of massage, they may be less familiar with specific sports and how to use these skills with athletes. Alternately, professionals such as athletic trainers and physical therapists who work with athletes may lack understanding of the physiological effects of manual therapy techniques and how to use them effectively in the context needed for their patients. In addition, many other professionals, including strength and conditioning coaches, may provide direction on recovery modalities (e.g., foam rolling) or look to work on mobility with their clients but lack the background of massage therapists, athletic trainers, and physical therapists. This book aims to fill these gaps for all professionals. It is not designed to be a step-by-step guide or how-to manual. Each profession, as well as each professional, has their own unique clinical perspective.

With this book, the hope is to unravel some of the mystery behind what is being done during manual therapy so practitioners can make the best decisions for their clients. *The Anatomy and Physiology of Sports Massage* answers questions regarding both why and what to do and why. Manual therapies are only as good as their therapeutic rationale. Most of the techniques presented here rely on treating the myofascial system but in context with the circulatory and nervous systems, especially the autonomic nervous system. It is easy to talk about homeostasis—or balance; but it is more difficult to create balance when sports themselves create imbalances in systems. People often ask me to "show them a thing or two," so they can learn what to do for sports massage. My response is always to hesitate: I know they do not know why they are doing what they are doing, and therein lies the problem. To paraphrase one of my mentors, massage is not just about "touching people." Massage is about the power of the touch and how it translates.

Part I, Foundations, addresses the why of sports massage. It reviews anatomy and physiology and describes how it relates to manual therapy (chapters 1 and 2), introduces massage techniques (chapter 3), and discusses structural versus functional considerations (chapter 4) and common compensations (chapter 5) found in sport. The information in part I is helpful for clinicians who want to know more about the why behind manual therapy techniques, for clinicians who are doing things because that is how they were told to do them, and for clinicians faced with the challenge of the patient asking for a treatment that does not match the goals of the session. As clinicians read about why specific manual therapies are used maybe more than once, they can realize the importance of the why: Why are clinicians using this technique? Why is this muscle reacting to the stress placed on it? Why are there trigger points here? Why focus on the sympathetic response of the body instead of the parasympathetic? There are so many reasons to ask "Why?"

Part II, Techniques, illustrates the what of sports massage. Manual therapy techniques are presented for specific muscles (chapters 6-10), and self-care is also discussed (chapter 11). The what of sports massage starts with the anatomy, or clinicians knowing what they are working with: What muscles are being stressed by the activity? What are clinicians feeling under their hands (or forearms or fingers) when they work? What treatments can clinicians do for the muscles to alleviate the muscles' stressors? Part II focuses on further understanding the why of sports massage and what to do with that information.

My hope is that whether the reader is a seasoned clinician, a clinical instructor, an educator, or a student, they can find some valuable foundations and techniques here to help treat the person on their table. For clinicians, having permission to put their hands on a patient and making a difference is a privilege. Plus, the human body is amazing. I hope you can appreciate it as much as I do.

PART I

Foundations

Part I explores the foundations of providing a sports massage treatment. Whether clinicians are developing a one-time treatment or creating a treatment plan, part I describes the why of the treatment: Why choose a particular type of treatment? Why will the chosen treatment be appropriate for the goals? Why are the stressors from a particular sport occurring?

Chapter 1 reviews the myofascial unit, muscle contraction, and physiology principles. Chapter 2 discusses the circulatory systems, somatic nervous system, and autonomic nervous system, in relation to why they are influenced by massage therapy. Chapter 3 reviews the principles of massage, including types of treatment and how they are intertwined with the physiological effects. Finally, chapters 4 and 5 discuss some common conditions practitioners may find in working with athletes or any active individuals who can benefit from sports massage.

The purpose of part I is to outline the background information before discussing any treatments found in part II. Some of the information here may be a review, whereas other information may be new, depending on the clinician's area of expertise. Regardless, part I can serve as background to help clinicians develop the goals of treatment and create a plan for their athletes.

Muscles and Fascia

Much of what is presented in this text can be found in numerous anatomy books. So how is this book different? This comprehensive resource aims to help clinicians increase their understanding of anatomy and physiology before they apply manual therapy concepts in the clinical context, even if the information itself is a review. This chapter reviews muscles and fascial structures and describes their importance in developing effective manual therapy treatments.

The *myofascial system* is the integral focus of any manual therapy treatment. In a simplified version of anatomy, fascia makes up the framework of the body, and muscles produce the movement. However, their interconnected relationship is more complex, because fascia is interwoven into the muscles. Better understanding of the relationship between muscles and their surrounding fascial layers helps clinicians apply the appropriate manual therapy treatments for the desired outcome. The *myofascial unit* integrates the muscles and fascia with the accessory structures of the connective tissue, nerves, and vessels and creates the interconnection where fascial disorders begin (Stecco et al. 2023). When fascia adheres to muscle, the muscle's ability to function properly can be compromised; such adherence can lead to insufficient blood flow, because local blood vessels may be compressed. In turn, the ability of the contractile portion of the muscle to perform also may be compromised, leading to inefficiency. Although it is not as simple as the clinician applying manual therapy techniques to improve muscle function, treatments become more effective with correct understanding of the myofascial system and the demands of physical training (Stecco et al. 2023).

Muscle and Fascia Connection

Each muscle is composed of muscle fibers (or cells) surrounded by a layer of fascia termed the *endomysium*, which is continuous with the cell membrane (or *sarcolemma*) (figure 1.1). Muscle fibers are unique in that they run from tendon to tendon in the body, meaning the cells of the muscles do not look like the pictures of round, small cells that readers may have studied in basic biology; rather, these cells are long, thin structures. Muscle fibers are then bundled in groups known as *fascicles*, which are surrounded by another layer of fascia termed the *perimysium*. Groups of fascicles make up the muscle belly, which is surrounded by a layer of fascia referred to as the *epimysium*.

The deep fascial layer of the body continues the myofascial connection as it surrounds various groups of muscles, such as the abdominal fascia and the fascia lata of the thigh. These groups can serve as muscle attachments as well as supportive structures. The deep fascia serves as an anchor for a small percentage of fascicles and as a link with the intermuscular connections. Fascia serves as a pathway for some of the force transmission generated by the muscles, assisting the tendons and bones (Stecco et al. 2023). Because manual therapies cannot truly reach these inner layers of the fascia, this interconnected network allows for the

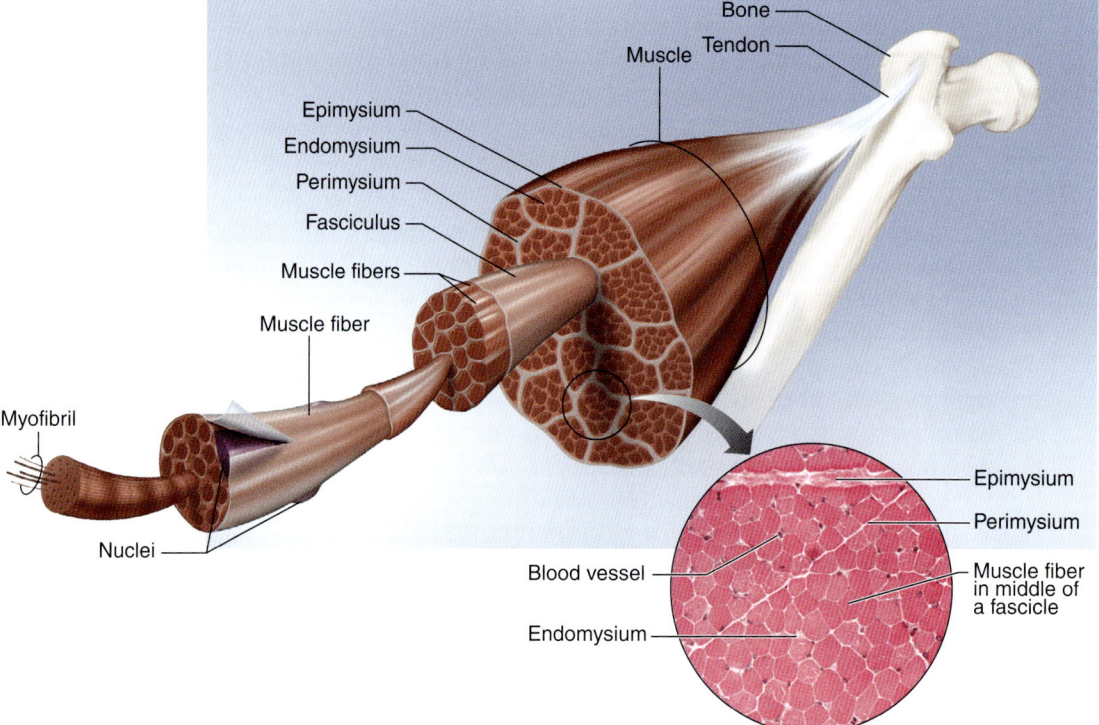

Figure 1.1 The muscle fibers become fascicles, the fascicles become muscle bellies, and the entire structure becomes part of the myofascial unit.

feeling of release deeper down by relieving the upper layers. Getting deep with massage is not so much a matter of pressure but of being smart and patient while working through the tissue layers.

Fascial Roles

Fascia plays a variety of roles in the body. *Dynamic fascia*, such as the thoracolumbar fascia, plays a role in movement and stability (Kumka and Bonar 2012). *Passive fascia* maintains continuity, allowing for force transmission and communication throughout the body. For example, the bicipital aponeurosis serves as an attachment for the biceps brachii (Kumka and Bonar 2012). *Compressive fascia* provides compression and tension, influencing venous return and enhancing muscular efficiency, coordination, and proprioception (Kumka and Bonar 2012). An example is the fascia lata that surrounds the thigh and provides efficiency to the quadriceps, hamstrings, and adductor muscle groups. *Separating fascia* creates compartments in the body to provide support, absorb shock, and maintain structural function. While separating fascia is mostly found as *parietal fascia* (lining the walls of body cavities) and *visceral fascia* (surrounding the internal organs)—treatment areas out of the scope of this text—the investing fascia of the abdomen is a relevant structure to manual therapy treatments (Kumka and Bonar 2012).

Fascial Response to Stress

The continuous nature of fascia creates a tension network that responds to the properties of *tensegrity*, which is a blend of tension and integrity. In anatomy, tensegrity occurs where there is a balance between the structural stability and compression of the bone and the dynamic balance of the tensioned soft tissues. To create balance in the body, when one part of the fascia is exposed to stress, another part will respond in opposition to maintain the tensegrity of the overall structure. *Stress* is defined as the load over the area, and *strain* is the change in shape as a result of the stress. Over time, the continued stress will lead to continued deformation, which can then result in a change in shape. Although fascia can return to its normal state when the stress is removed, too much time under the influence of the stress will lead to a permanent change to the myofascial unit.

Consider the example of athletes who have spent many hours at their sport over many years: Their bodies adapt to the stresses put on the tissues. With the correct combination of manual therapy, stretching, and strengthening, clinicians do their best to work within clients' limitations. As described in chapter 4, sometimes clinicians cannot completely eradicate these changes, but they can work with them to create as much balance as possible throughout the body.

Fascia responds to stress by shortening, solidifying, and thickening, which is also referred to as *binding down*. Stress can lead to biomechanical inefficiency and greater energy consumption. Restrictions in fascia during the stress spread through the structures, leading to a loss of flexibility and spontaneity of movement. These restrictions can form through the area of an injury and throughout the associated *fascial lines*, the interconnected pathways of the connective tissue. For example, changes in the gastrocnemius and the soleus complex may lead to issues in the plantar fascia, and restrictions in the thoracolumbar fascia may alter movement of the shoulder through the latissimus dorsi. From a treatment perspective, it is important for clinicians not to have a singular focus and to look beyond the area of concern (proximal or distal) when needed. For example, fascial issues near the knee could be coming from the hip, the foot, or both.

Fascia can be influenced by a variety of internal and external factors, some of which the patient may have control over and others which they may not. Trauma, whether physical or emotional, can negatively affect fascia. Although physical trauma, such as injury, is in the scope of the health care professionals for whom this book is written, emotional trauma is not, and appropriate referrals should be made as necessary. Acute or overuse injuries are related to fascial changes, either causing the changes or resulting from issues in the fascial system. Emotional stress can also be a factor, because stress often causes the body to feel tight, with this tightness coming from the muscles or the fascial structures. Inflammation as a response to injury, a medical condition, or medication also can influence the fascia. It is important to obtain a thorough patient medical history to identify any potential cautions or contraindications before beginning any manual therapy (see chapter 3). Another major influence on the fascia are common adaptations, either for sport or for postural habits, which are covered in chapter 5.

Relevant Fascial Structures

Although fascia is continuous throughout the body, certain structures receive a bit more tension and notoriety than others (figure 1.2). Typically, the iliotibial (IT) band and the plantar fascia are considered relevant fascial structures; however, these structures do not exist in isolation. The IT band overlaps the fascia lata surrounding the thigh. Think of the fascia lata as plastic wrap surrounding the thigh muscles, with the IT band as the overlap of the ends to seal off the thigh. The plantar fascia starts at the calcaneal tubercle, which is the ultimate insertion of the Achilles tendon, the common tendon for the gastrocnemius and the soleus. Therefore, any injury or shortening of the gastrocnemius and the soleus can pull on the plantar fascia. From a treatment perspective, clinicians must pay attention to all areas where the structures meet and meld. If clinicians treat only one area and ignore the structures above and below on the kinetic chain, they may miss a chance to create an effective treatment.

Common Fascial Structures

A list of common fascial structures is provided next. Although this list is not exhaustive, these structures are commonly seen as having dysfunction related to overuse in sports.

- *Iliotibial band.* This structure overlaps the fascia lata at the distal lateral aspect of the thigh. The IT band serves as the insertion of the tensor fasciae latae on the lateral tibia at Gerdy's tubercle. A portion of the gluteus maximus also inserts into the IT band.
- *Fascia lata.* This deep fascia of the thigh surrounds the quadriceps, hamstring, and adductor muscle groups.
- *Plantar fascia* (figure 1.2a). This structure is found on the plantar surface of the foot, and it runs from the calcaneal tubercle to the toes. The plantar fascia has many layers and is more complex than just a strip of connective tissue. The central part is thicker, creating the plantar aponeurosis, whereas the medial and lateral parts are weaker.
- *Thoracolumbar fascia* (figure 1.2b). This multilayered structure is found in the lower back, the white triangle, as an attachment for muscles of the glenohumeral joint (latissimus dorsi), the abdomen (transversus abdominis), the low back (multifidus), and the gluteal region (gluteus maximus). The thoracolumbar fascia is a fascial stress point, because there are multiple muscles pulling in varying directions from this region. One of the three layers of the thoracolumbar fascia is the thoracolumbar aponeurosis, the posterior layer that serves as a site for muscle attachment.
- *Bicipital aponeurosis.* This structure is the fascial connection of the biceps brachii to the ulna, which also covers the cubital fossa.
- *Pectoral fascia.* This structure covers the pectoralis major, becoming continuous with the anterior abdominal wall distally and the axillary fascia laterally.

Less Common Fascial Structures

The following structures may not be the first that come to mind when considering fascial structures. However, they provide support to the movements of the body and can be subjected to the same stresses of the more common structures.

- *Retinaculum* (figure 1.2c). This structure holds the tendons in place, ensuring a correct line of pull for biomechanical efficiency. Although the retinacula are described in textbooks as distinct structures, examinations of this structure in cadavers indicate that the retinacula are part of the deep fascia.
- *Inguinal ligament* (figure 1.2d). This ligament runs from the pubic tubercle to the anterior superior iliac spine. It is a crease formed at the meeting of the abdominal fascia and the fascia lata.
- *Crural fascia.* This structure is the deep fascia found in the lower leg. It forms the intermuscular septa that create the compartments in the lower leg.
- *Interosseous membranes.* These membranes serve as muscle attachments for two main interosseous membranes that sit between the radius and the ulna as well as the tibia and the fibula.

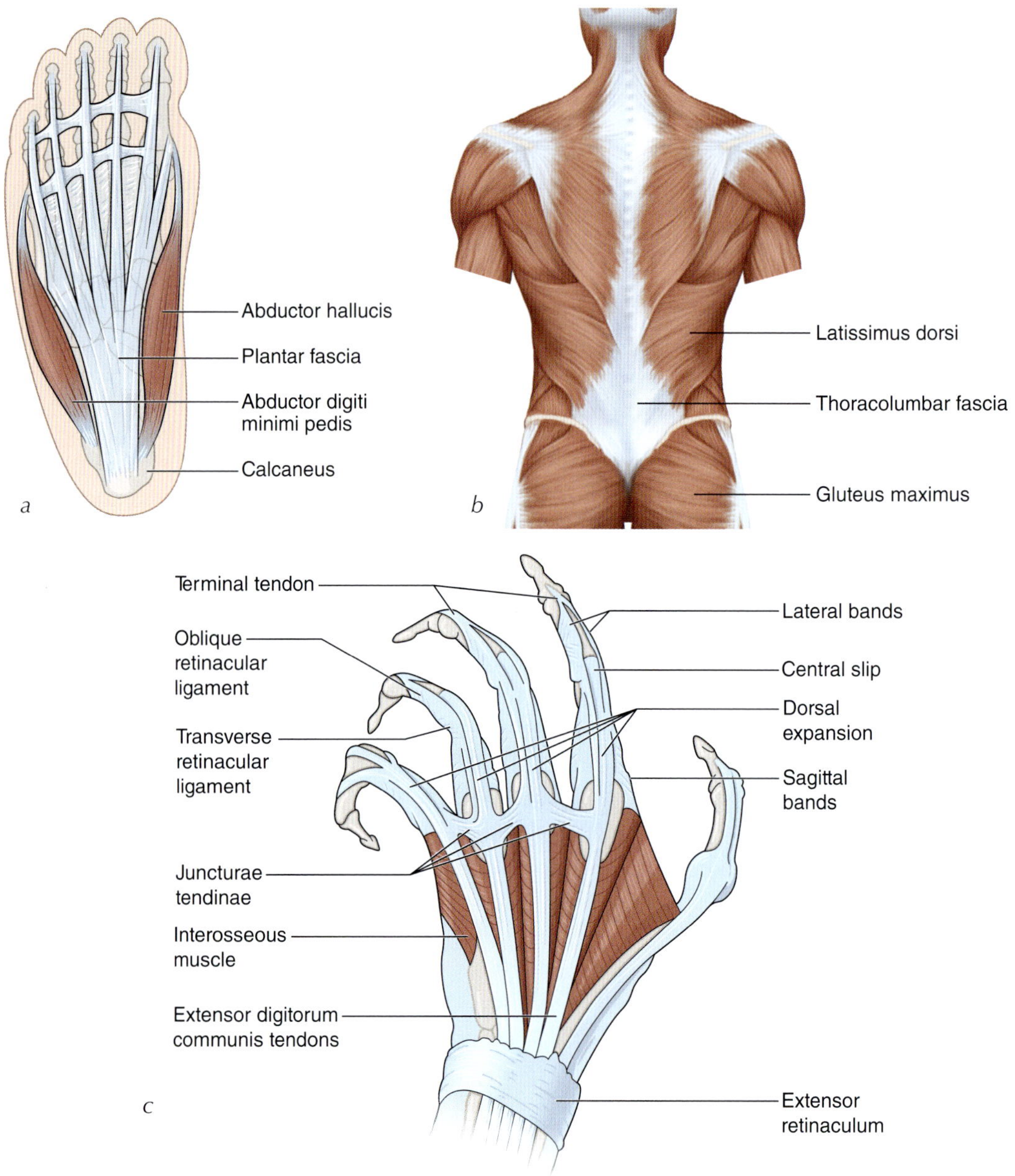

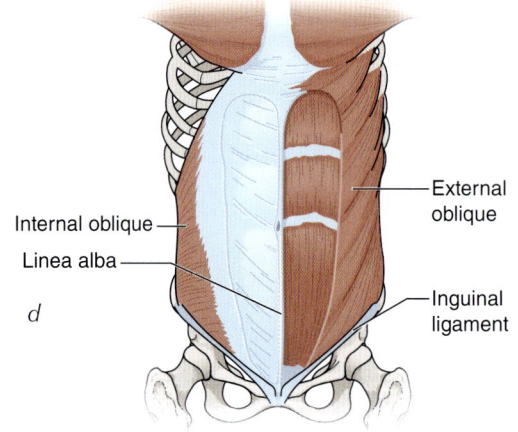

Figure 1.2 (a) The plantar fascia from the calcaneus to the toes, (b) the thoracolumbar fascia as it connects to the latissimus dorsi and gluteus maximus, (c) the extensor retinaculum that serves to maintain the anatomical pull of the finger extensor muscles, and (d) the abdominal fascia (bottom right) with the abdominal muscles, its midline attachment of the linea alba, and the inferior attachment to the inguinal ligament.

Muscles

There are three types of muscle in the body: cardiac, smooth, and skeletal. *Cardiac muscle* is striated, is involuntary, and is found only in the heart. *Smooth muscle* is not striated, is involuntary, and is found in the organs. *Skeletal muscle* is striated and voluntary, attaching to the bones and producing movement at the joints. Muscles create movement, stabilize posture, assist with circulation, and produce heat as a byproduct of muscle contraction. Throughout this text, the term *muscle* will specifically refer to skeletal muscle unless noted otherwise.

Review of Muscle Basics

Properties of muscle tissue include excitability, contractility, extensibility, and elasticity. *Excitability* is the response of the muscle to stimuli; with sufficient stimuli, the muscle will respond by developing tension, which is *contractility*. *Extensibility* is the capacity of the muscle to stretch, and *elasticity* is the ability of the muscle to return to its original length after being stretched. As readers delve further into manual therapy, it is important to keep in mind these basic properties (see chapter 3).

When muscles develop tension, sometimes referred to as *muscle contraction*, the force produced results in muscle action. These actions will sometimes produce a change in the length of the muscle, causing changes to the position of bones and movement around the joint. Muscle actions that produce a change in length are *isotonic* (from ancient Greek roots *iso tonos*, meaning "equal tension"). These changes can result in either a shortening (*concentric*) or lengthening (*eccentric*) contraction. Not all contractions result in a change in length. *Isometric* (from ancient Greek roots *iso metron*, meaning "equal measure") contractions are tension in the muscle that does not result in a change in length. All types of contractions can be used to enhance a manual therapy treatment.

Muscle contractions are initiated by the motor nerves to the muscles fibers they innervate. The motor nerve and the fibers they innervate are known as the *motor unit*, and one branch of a motor nerve innervates a number of muscle fibers. When the brain signals to a motor nerve that a contraction should be initiated, the motor nerve releases acetylcholine at its attachment to the muscle. The presence of acetylcholine signals the fiber to initiate the muscle contraction. A muscle fiber contracts under the all-or-none principle, in which the fiber contracts completely or not at all. What makes a contraction stronger is the number of motor units that are recruited, not the strength of the recruitment. For example, if someone picks up this book, their brain might recruit 5 motor units; but if they pick up a 20-pound dumbbell, their brain would recruit 50 motor units.

Muscles play a variety of roles when moving the body. The primary mover of an action or the muscle of reference (i.e., the muscle the clinician is focused on at the time) is the *agonist* (e.g., biceps brachii as an elbow flexor). Muscles that assist the agonist, providing the same action, are the *synergists* (e.g., the synergist to the biceps brachii would be the brachialis, also an elbow flexor). Muscles that produce the opposite action are *antagonists* (e.g., the triceps brachii, an elbow extensor, is the antagonist to the biceps brachii). Muscles that hold the area in a neutral position during contraction are *neutralizers* (e.g., when holding the forearm in a supinated position, the supinator would serve as a neutralizer). Finally, muscles that support structures to prevent excessive motion are *stabilizers* (e.g., the rhomboids help to stabilize the scapula, which is the proximal attachment for the biceps brachii).

Knowing the terminology helps with muscle treatment, as will be discussed in the Physiology Rules section of this chapter. To create balance in the body, clinicians may consider treating the antagonist to promote function in the agonist (e.g., strengthening one and stretching the other). They also need to consider the role of the stabilizers and neutralizers because if they are not working correctly, the agonist may not be able to provide the most efficient line of pull. Understanding the role the muscle plays in the dysfunction can help create an optimal treatment.

Muscle Shapes, Arrangements, and Nomenclature

The shape and the fiber arrangement of muscles are related to their ability to produce force and to exert that force through a range of motion. As mentioned earlier, muscle fibers run between tendons. The longer the muscle fiber, the more its primary function is range of motion; the shorter the fiber, the more its primary function is force production. The arrangement of the fibers helps determine the function of the muscle, with some muscles having a combination of fiber arrangements. Muscle fibers arranged in a parallel fashion include

- flat (muscles that are broad and thin),
- fusiform (muscles shaped with a central belly that tapers at each end),
- strap (muscles that are long and thin),
- radiate (muscles that are a fan-shaped combination of thin and fusiform), and
- sphincter (muscles that are round).

Pennate muscles have fibers arranged like a feather with oblique lines to the tendon. The three types of pennate muscles are named according to their arrangement from the tendon:

- Unipennate (run from one side of the tendon only)
- Bipennate (run from both sides of the tendon)
- Multipennate (several tendons with fibers running diagonally between them)

When learning or remembering muscles, it is best to understand the categories by which muscles can be named:

- Size (gluteus maximus, gluteus minimus, adductor longus, and adductor brevis)
- Location (rectus abdominis, peroneus longus, and pectoralis major)

- Shape (teres major, trapezius, and rhomboid major)
- Actions performed (extensor digitorum longus, flexor hallucis longus, and supinator)
- Attachments (brachioradialis)
- Fiber direction (internal obliques or rectus femoris)

Muscles can be named with any of the combinations just described. Associating the muscles with the different ways of creating their names while thinking of anatomy as its own language makes the learning process easier over time.

Muscles have two areas of attachment to the bones via tendons. One attachment is *proximal*, considered the *origin*, which is typically stable during contraction. The other attachment is *distal*, considered the *insertion*, which typically moves toward the origin during contraction. The tendons that attach muscle to bone are made up of the *epimysium fascia* surrounding the muscle and blend into the *periosteum*, which surrounds the bones.

Sliding Filament Theory and Muscle Contractions

Muscle fibers are made up of smaller myofibrils, which are divided into sections termed *sarcomeres* and are composed of myofilaments (figure 1.3). *Myofilaments*

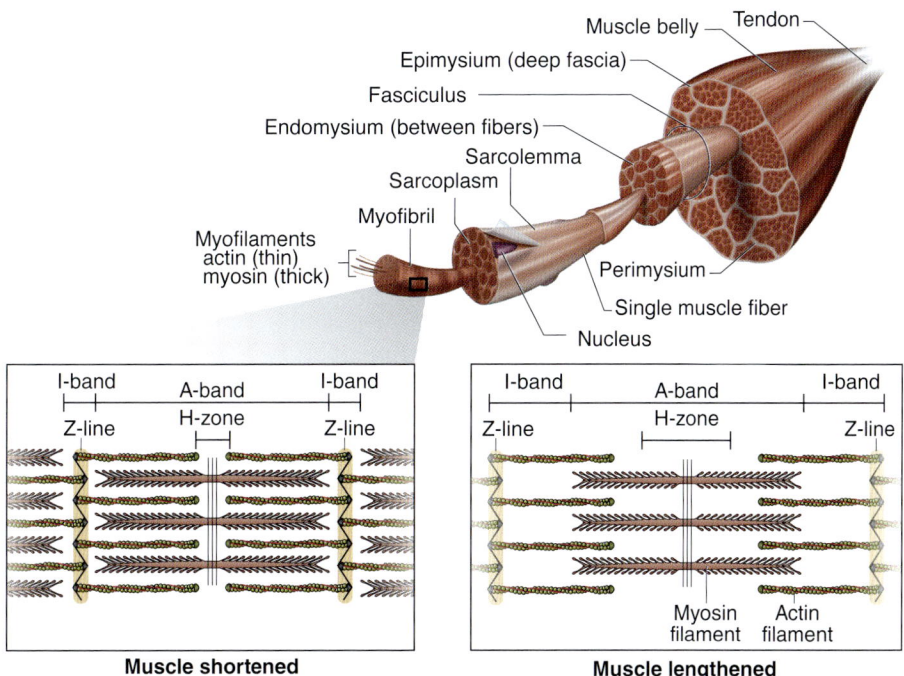

Figure 1.3 The illustration shows a shortened (concentric) and lengthened (eccentric) contraction using the sliding filament theory.

are composed of the thick filaments made up of myosin and the thin filaments consist of actin. The thin filaments are anchored to the z lines creating the sarcomere (sarcomeres run from z line to z line). *Myosin* contains heads branching off the thick filament, whereas *actin* contains binding sites covered by tropomyosin molecules, held in place by troponin, preventing the myosin heads from binding with the actin. When calcium is introduced to the area, the binding sites open, allowing for the contraction cycle to begin. There is a ratcheting effect of the myosin heads pulling on the thin filaments, bringing the z lines closer together. This effect continues as long as the binding sites are open and energy (in the form of adenosine triphosphate, ATP) is present.

During the contraction cycle, the z lines move closer together. If the z lines get close enough, the muscle will shorten (concentric contraction). If the muscle stimulation is not enough to produce force but is not shortening, an isometric contraction will occur. Furthermore, if the contraction is such to increase the joint angle, an eccentric contraction will occur and the muscle will lengthen. Should the calcium remain, the binding sites will be open, and the contraction will be sustained. This description is a bit of an oversimplification of the more complex process, but it provides enough of a review of the physiology involved to put things in perspective for the scope of this book.

Postural and Phasic Muscles

Muscles are identified as either postural or phasic based on their function, location, and response to stress. Some muscles may be classified as both because they have multiple parts that act antagonistically (e.g., the trapezius, specifically the upper and lower portions), muscle groups that cross multiple joints (e.g., proximal and distal hamstrings), or muscles that can react differently based on their fiber directions and the stresses put on them (e.g., infraspinatus and latissimus dorsi). During training, muscles adapt in relation to the stresses put on them. This adaptation is one of the goals of training. However, some positive adaptations for a sport may lead to negative adaptations on the contralateral side or with the antagonistic muscles. For example, bench press is a great exercise for building up the anterior aspect of the torso; however, shortening of the pectoralis major can lead to eccentric strain on the middle trapezius and the rhomboids. Realizing where the adaptation will occur and what stress on a particular muscle will look like is the first part to a successful treatment.

POSTURAL MUSCLES
Postural muscles support the body against gravity. Typically, postural muscles are composed of more slow-twitch fibers; they are aerobic based in their use of energy, meaning they tend to have higher amounts of small blood vessels; and they are fatigue resistant (Chaitow and DeLany 2000). Postural muscles are responsible for fine-tuning movements to maintain the center of gravity over the base of support. However, the fine-tuning movements may lead to limitations in the mobility of the muscle. Postural muscles therefore respond to stress by

shortening and contracting, as they are charged with compensating for misalignment in the joints.

It is important not to confuse a muscle shortening and contracting with the presence of strength. Postural muscles may appear strong or weak with manual muscle testing. Because of their positioning in relation to the bony landmarks, they may not be able to produce a strong contraction if they lose their biomechanical advantage. Also, the muscle fibers may be in a state of hypertonicity, in which the fibers are already contracted and unavailable for additional contraction (Chaitow and DeLany 2000).

PHASIC MUSCLES

Phasic muscles move the body through gravity. Typically, phasic muscles have more fast-twitch fibers, and they are more anaerobic based in their use of energy. They are quick to respond with more powerful contraction, but they fatigue more easily. Phasic muscles respond to stress by lengthening and weakening. At times, they may become inhibited and unable to perform their functions in neutral positions. As phasic muscles become lengthened, the body lays down more connective tissue to maintain the integrity between bony landmarks (see chapter 4). Fascia binds to support where muscles cannot. This connective tissue lacks the ability to contract, thereby further weakening the muscle. Often, phasic muscles are a source of pain resulting from the stress or pull of the muscles, and individuals will feel that they need to stretch; however, it is important to avoid lengthening muscle that is already in a lengthened state.

Physiology Rules

Muscle and fascial physiology have a few rules for clinicians to consider as they build treatments and use the techniques presented in chapter 3. These principles will guide clinicians in responding to the different dysfunctions presented.

Davis' Law

The introduction of mechanical stimulation to tissues leads to remodeling (Loghmani and Whitted 2016). When applied to soft tissue, this is known as *Davis' law*. What makes this law interesting in the context of manual therapy is its effect in the direction of causing some level of dysfunction as well as relieving the dysfunction. The training an athlete undergoes, as well as the individual's activities of daily living and habits, can lead to changes in the soft tissue structure. The application of manual therapy, along with stretching and strengthening, can be used to cause change that can alleviate pain and dysfunction.

In applying Davis' law to a postural muscle, which responds by shortening, the body will remove tissue to keep the same congruency between bony landmarks. Think about the pectoralis minor (see chapter 6), a protractor of the scapula: As it shortens in response to stress, the coracoid process (the insertion) will position itself closer to the ribs (the origin on ribs three through five). Prolonged time in this position will result in the tissue being removed, effectively moving the scapula further from the spine on the posterior view and bringing it more anterior around the ribs. Because the muscle always runs from one bony landmark to another, shortening of the muscle results in a repositioning of the bones.

With a phasic muscle, such as the rhomboids, the opposite result is seen with Davis' law. The rhomboids are scapular retractors, antagonists to the pectoralis minor. As the scapula moves laterally from the spine, the insertion of the rhomboids (the medial border of the scapula) becomes further from the origin (the spinous processes of C7 to T5). In response, the body lays down more connective tissue to lengthen the muscle. Chapters 6 to 10 in part II of this book focus on specific muscles, and they further discuss how these dysfunctions can lead to issues and, more importantly, how manual therapy can be used to work through them.

Postisometric Relaxation

Following an isometric contraction of a muscle, it will relax more fully. This rule can be used in a variety of ways in life as well as in massage. For example, if a muscle is feeling tight or has a cramp, then contracting that muscle causes it to relax more fully. This technique is referred to as *postisometric relaxation*, and it can also be used to relieve emotional tension. Consider this example: Do you find that your shoulders elevate toward your ears while you are reading all this information? Contract your upper trapezius and levator scapulae. Now release. Did you feel it? Has that tension diminished? That is postisometric relaxation: It has not only a physical effect but also an emotional one.

The concept of postisometric relaxation can be used in manual therapy by bringing a muscle to the barrier of its stretch, releasing back from that position, and having the patient isometrically contract the muscle just enough to elicit a response. Once the muscle relaxes, the stretch barrier will be increased, producing a greater range of motion. Although this technique is typically used for stretching, it can also be used to assist with greater relaxation of the muscles during a massage session. By combining this physiology rule with the techniques in chapter 3, clinicians can assist clients in lengthening a postural muscle.

Reciprocal Inhibition

With *reciprocal inhibition*, contraction of the antagonist will lead to relaxation of the agonist as the reciprocal muscle of the one being contracted becomes inhibited. Because only one muscle (agonist or antagonist) can be contracted at a time, the clinician can force the relaxation of the agonist without having that muscle contract. This rule can be used the same as with postisometric relaxation, just initiating different muscles, which is beneficial when the patient cannot contract the muscle being treated. As with postisometric relaxation, reciprocal inhibition can be used to stretch the agonist or to soften a muscle to apply a treatment. Here is another example of how to use this technique: If you have cramps in the gastrocnemius (a plantar flexor), then initiating contraction of the tibialis anterior (a dorsiflexor) will cause the gastrocnemius to relax more fully. This technique can be used by someone having calf cramps in the middle of the night. Activating the antagonist helps relieve the cramping.

Mechanoreceptors

Muscles and fascia have a variety of structures within them that allow for neural feedback, termed *mechanoreceptors*. These mechanoreceptors have a variety of functions, with the intent of interplaying between the muscle and the nervous system—the brains of the operation. The mechanoreceptors provide feedback about the position of the tissues and the joints, sending that information via sensory neurons to the central nervous system for interpretation. Mechanoreceptors from the somatic nervous system perspective are examined in chapter 2. This chapter examines them from the perspective of the muscles and the fascia.

Within the muscles are *muscle spindle fibers*, which have the primary role of monitoring not only the stretch of a muscle but also its rate of change in length. Should you attempt to stretch a muscle too far or too fast, the muscle spindle fibers signal the central nervous system, which responds by initiating a contraction of the muscle. Within the musculotendinous junction are *Golgi tendon organs* (GTOs) that monitor the tension in a muscle from either end. When there is too much tension in a muscle, the GTOs send signals to the central nervous system and respond by relaxing the muscle. Because their response is related to tension, GTOs only respond to active stretching; passive stretches will not elicit a response. Together, the muscle spindle fibers and GTOs work in opposition, but the result prevents muscle damage from either overstretching or excess tension.

Two mechanoreceptors take center stage in monitoring the position of the joints. The *Ruffini organs*, found in ligaments and outer capsule layers, and *Pacinian corpuscles*, found in deeper capsular layers and more distal aspects of the tendons, monitor the tissue changes around the joints, relaying information to the nervous system. The Pacinian corpuscles respond to rapid pressure changes and vibrations, but they shut down soon after the movement stops. High-velocity thrusts activate a response from the Pacinian corpuscles (Schleip 2003a). The Ruffini organs detect slower change around a joint's position, specifically responding to tangential forces and sustained pressure (Schleip 2003a). The Ruffini organs are slower to adapt, and they continue to send signals even after the stimulus stops. The response of these mechanoreceptors to stimulation is part of the reason why manual therapy, specifically the use of myofascial treatments, is effective in eliciting change to the tissue.

WHY DOES THE CLINICIAN CARE?

Understanding how muscles work within the body and how they respond to stress can help clinicians create a correct treatment plan. For example, many people with upper back pain (rhomboids or middle trapezius area) will be inclined to stretch. However, because these are phasic muscles, they are already lengthened. By knowing that the anterior chest is the antagonist (I see you, pectoralis major), which is postural and likely to be shortened, clinicians can better treat upper back pain with a nice stretch to open the anterior chest. With understanding of concepts such as postisometric relaxation or reciprocal inhibition, clinicians can work with the muscles in pairs as either agonist and synergist or agonist and antagonist.

With sports in which a client may have muscle asymmetry because of the use of a dominant side (right or left), clinicians would follow similar treatment objectives but work one side of the body differently from the other. For example, a tennis player or baseball pitcher may have a stronger right side compared with the left, whereas a dancer may have an imbalance between the leg used to take off compared with the leg used for landing. The overpowering of one side versus another could lead to dysfunction in other areas of the kinetic chain. Although clinicians do not want the patient to lose the strength and power of the involved side, they need to work on balance to make the patient's body as efficient as possible.

With the muscles on the axial skeleton, the antagonist to a muscle could be the same muscle on the opposite side. Imagine using the right and left external obliques of the abdomen while doing a rotational movement, such as hitting a baseball or swinging a golf club. In this example, there are different adaptations to each side, and the clinician needs to treat them accordingly. Just as clinicians would need to treat the pectoralis minor to find relief in the rhomboids, they would need to treat the left and right external obliques differently because with a right-handed swing the right side would respond as a postural muscle, whereas the left side would be the phasic muscle.

The remainder of part I reviews the physiological effects of manual therapies (chapter 2), describes the types of manual therapies (chapter 3), and discusses structural and functional considerations (chapter 4) and common stressors in sport (chapter 5). In part II, chapters 6 to 10 outline techniques specific to individual muscles. When clinicians combine all of this knowledge with understanding of the daily stressors facing their patient, they can better create an individualized treatment.

The Physiological Effects of Manual Therapies

One of the greatest clinical application mismatches is between the intent of treatment and the type of treatment selected. Many times, I see clinicians choose massage strokes that they think are for circulatory purposes but do not, in fact, influence fluid movement, or they create a treatment that promotes a parasympathetic response before a practice or game. There are a variety of reasons for these mismatches: Some clinicians only use the tools they know, others use anecdotal evidence (i.e., what someone told them, without checking sources), and others do what the client asks even if their request is incorrect. Even with the research available, much of the information is not straightforward.

The use of evidence-informed practice is paramount, but the evidence will not tell clinicians what to do directly. There are other considerations: What is the response of the organ system the clinician is influencing? What are the goals of the session? Does the treatment match the goals?

This chapter reviews the various body systems, and it describes purported physiological responses to the manual therapy treatments outlined in chapter 3. For clinicians, creating a treatment plan balances the techniques they know, the response of the body, and the goals of the patient, combined with timing, anatomy, and other variables.

Circulatory Systems

The *circulatory systems* are responsible for the movement of fluid through the vessels. The cardiovascular system comprises the heart and blood vessels and is a closed system, whereas the lymphatic system is an open system. The lymphatic system is responsible for fluid return only, whereas the circulatory system is responsible for both fluid distribution and return. Although fluid movement through the cardiovascular system is initiated by the heart, fluid return in both systems is influenced by movement. Contraction of the skeletal muscles assists in pushing fluid from both systems back to the heart. Additionally, deep diaphragmatic breaths can help to guide lymphatic return from the lower extremity and venous return in the thoracic cavity by changes in intrathoracic pressure. Massage is highly recognized for its physiological influence on the movement of fluid through the vessels. The research has reported varying results as to whether this influence is related more to the manual movement of blood or to changes in pressure resulting from technique application (Moraska 2005).

Cardiovascular System

The *cardiovascular system* is a closed system that moves blood through the network of vessels and back to the heart. Systemic effects of circulatory massage on the cardiovascular system include decreased heart rate and blood pressure (Cambron et al. 2006). Locally, massage increases blood flow to the treatment area, which is associated with increased oxygen, nutrients, and histamine. Fluid movement may also allow for removal of noxious chemicals that lead to painful sensations associated with delayed-onset muscle soreness (Moraska 2005). Many systemic effects of massage are further influenced by autonomic nervous system response, in which the vagus nerve (cranial nerve X) initiates heart rate changes via the parasympathetic pathways (Resnick 2016).

The heart is a double pump, moving blood from the upper chambers (*atria*) to the lower chambers (*ventricles*). When blood returns to the heart via the vena cava, it is pumped from the right atrium through the tricuspid valve to the right ventricle (figure 2.1). From the right ventricle, blood moves through the pulmonary valve into the pulmonary arteries to the lungs, where gas exchange occurs. The now-oxygenated blood returns to the left atrium via the pulmonary veins, and it is pumped through the mitral (bicuspid) valve into the left ventricle. The left ventricle is responsible for pumping blood through the aortic valve into the aorta, where it moves through the vascular network. Blood flows in the following order: from the aorta to the arteries, arterioles, capillaries, venules, veins, and vena cava and then back to the heart.

On a local level, compression of the tissues helps push blood through the venous system. In addition to the mechanical movement of fluid, compression alters the pressure in the veins; this change in pressure encourages fluid movement. Additionally, joint movement, both passive and active, encourages fluid movement. Therefore, even when the manual therapy treatment includes passive movements by clinicians, venous return is encouraged.

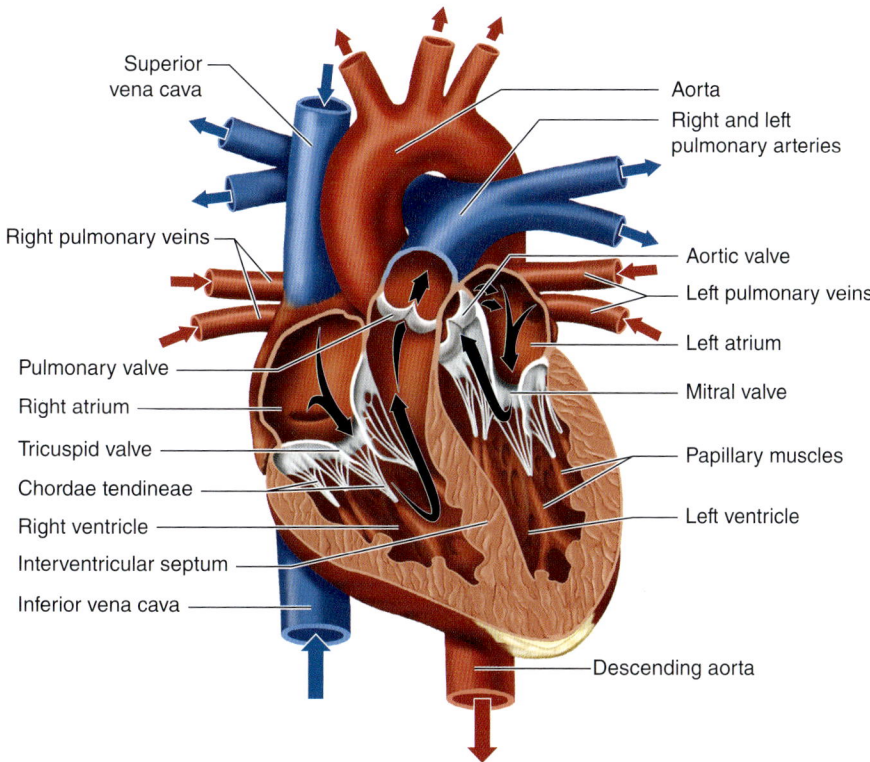

Figure 2.1 Blood flow through the heart. The black arrows trace the pathway of the blood through the heart from the right atrium to the right ventricle to the lungs. The now-oxygenated blood goes from the left atrium to the left ventricle, where it is pumped to the rest of the body.

Several sports massage techniques encourage active movements, as described in chapter 3.

Massage stimulates the release of histamine, which chemically encourages vasodilation. By expanding the lumen of the blood vessels, more blood can reach the affected tissues. The greater the blood supply, the more available oxygen and nutrients and the more efficient the metabolic waste removal. The chemical response of histamine has a circulatory component but also interfaces with the autonomic nervous system response, resulting in dilation or constriction of the blood vessels through pathways to maintain homeostasis. Although these are not direct circulatory effects, they are indirect changes to the cardiovascular network.

There is little agreement from the literature in regard to the influence of massage on the larger blood vessels. Many of the main arteries are situated close to the bone and inaccessible to direct stimulation. The more superficial arteries—such as the femoral artery in the femoral triangle, the popliteal artery in the popliteal space, and the brachial artery on the medial aspect of the arm—require caution when proceeding with treatment. The superficial arteries can be very sensitive, and practitioners should avoid applying excessive pressure during massage to prevent occluding the artery. However, as with the fascia, manipulation to the more superficial layers can cascade down to affect these vessels. Typically, in massage, the movement of fluid is encouraged toward the heart to assist the veins; because of the heart's pumping action, the arteries do not need assistance in moving blood into the tissues. Vein walls have minimal amounts of smooth muscle, so the veins cannot directly push blood through the venous system. However, veins have one-way valves that stop backflow against gravity. Because veins are more superficial, they are under greater influence by manual therapy than the arteries; however, they are not as superficial as the lymphatic vessels found in the lymphatic system.

Lymphatic System

The *lymphatic system* is an open system of vessels not connected in a full circuit with each other or the heart. The lymphatic system provides fluid return only and can be thought of as the overflow system for interstitial fluid (figure 2.2). During normal cardiovascular circulation, blood leaks from the capillaries to bring nutrients and oxygen to the area. *Plasma*, the fluid portion of the blood, becomes interstitial fluid when it leaks from the capillaries. When the same fluid moves into the lymphatic vessels, it becomes *lymph*. Essentially, there is approximately 10 percent more fluid in the cardiovascular system than it can handle, and this excess is taken up by the lymphatic system. Because this fluid does not have its own pump (like the heart supplies to the cardiovascular system), it can become stagnant either in one area or throughout the body. Therapy techniques specific to the lymphatic system can be used to reduce or control secondary swelling (*edema*). This type of manual therapy requires very light touch in the direction of lymph flow.

The lymphatic system is made up of vessels with one-way valves, keeping fluid moving through the system from distal to proximal points on the body. The vessel walls are more permeable than capillaries, allowing fluid to enter easily. However, once inside the vessel, pressure changes occur to keep the fluid in the vessels while the one-way valves keep the fluid from

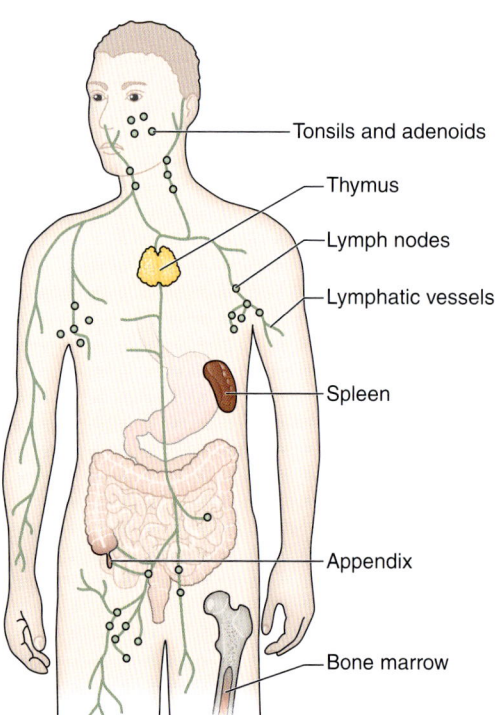

Figure 2.2 The lymphatic system is an open system of vessels that helps with the overflow of fluid outside the circulatory system.

reversing course. As the fluid moves proximally through the lymphatic system, the vessels become less permeable with walls that are less porous. Unlike the flow of the cardiovascular system through its network, the lymphatic system has more of a regional flow pattern with catchments for each specific group of vessels.

Normal fluid moves from the lymphatic system as follows. Fluid enters the lymphatic capillaries, which drain into the larger and less permeable lymphatic vessels. The lymphatic vessels converge into the larger trunks. On the right side of the upper body, the lymphatic trunk leads to the right lymphatic duct, which drains into the right subclavian vein on its return to the heart. The lymphatic trunks of the left side of the upper body join the lymphatic trunks of the entire lower body at the thoracic duct, which drains into the left subclavian vein. During its travels through the body, lymph passes through catchment areas and lymph node beds, where it is cleared of pathogens and abnormal cells. Any backups in this area may result in fluid stagnation and buildup.

There are a variety of lymphatic system treatments, including manual lymphatic drainage, lymphatic massage, and lymphedema techniques, all of which are outside the scope of this text. Techniques such as these require more advanced training, and there are many accomplished clinicians who can present such training. This book aims to introduce and increase clinicians' understanding of what is occurring physiologically. True lymphatic techniques are used to remove edema and to reduce or control secondary edema. These techniques also allow for protein uptake from the lymphatic system, and they serve to decrease any stagnancy that may occur. Additional cautions are needed for clients with pitting edema, those who have undergone lymph node removal as part of cancer staging, and those receiving chemotherapy. Again, these lymphatic techniques require specific training. For these populations, it is important to recognize the limitations of using the techniques presented in this book, and manual therapy treatment should be considered a contraindication unless the clinician is properly trained.

When performing any technique, the clinician should consider the location of the lymphatic vessels. These vessels are more superficial than the larger veins and arteries. Therefore, the massage techniques used to influence the lymphatic vessels must be very superficial, with light strokes in the direction of lymphatic flow. Passive movement can also encourage movement of lymph. Pressure that is too deep will not influence the lymphatic system; therefore, if the patient is seeking a lymphatic treatment, they should be informed that the use of excessive pressure is ill-advised. The intent with any lymphatic treatment is to stimulate uptake of edema, making appropriate use of pressure a must.

In the realm of sports massage, lymphatic facilitation can assist with removal of inflammation related to acute injury or surgery. The presence of excess fluid can hinder muscle range of motion and contractility. However, fluid serves a purpose as part of the healing process to clean up the injury site and begin to lay down new tissue. It is up to the clinician to balance the desired increase in strength and range of motion with the necessary physiological changes that occur as part of healing. These treatments cannot speed up the healing process, but they can be used to create an optimal environment for healing to occur.

Respiratory System

The *respiratory system* includes the nose, mouth, trachea, bronchi, larynx, and lungs as well as the diaphragm, which is the main muscle involved in breathing (figure 2.3). The diaphragm is a skeletal muscle, but breathing is a nonvoluntary action: People do not need to think about breathing, which is controlled by the respiratory center in the pons and the medulla oblongata of the brain stem. However, they can contract the diaphragm voluntarily to control their own breathing rate and depth.

During inhalation (*inspiration*), the diaphragm contracts and flattens. This contraction pushes the abdominal organs down, increasing the space in the thoracic cavity and decreasing the pressure in the lungs. As the pressure in the lungs decreases, air moves from a place of higher pressure (the atmosphere) to lower pressure (the lungs).

Exhalation (*expiration*) is a passive movement of air; when the diaphragm relaxes, the pressure in the lungs increases and air moves out to the atmosphere. Forced exhalation occurs when the abdominal muscles are contracted, pushing the abdominal contents up against the diaphragm, decreasing the space in the lungs, and forcing the air out. As noted earlier, the normal movement of air occurs such that people do not even consider breathing unless it is in dysfunction. However, dysfunctional breathing can lead to myofascial pain, and structural or functional concerns can lead to muscle dysfunction.

Breathing is often integrated with manual therapy because focused breathing has many advantages. Because changes in abdominal cavity pressure can help move fluid through venous return and lymphatic return, the breath can positively

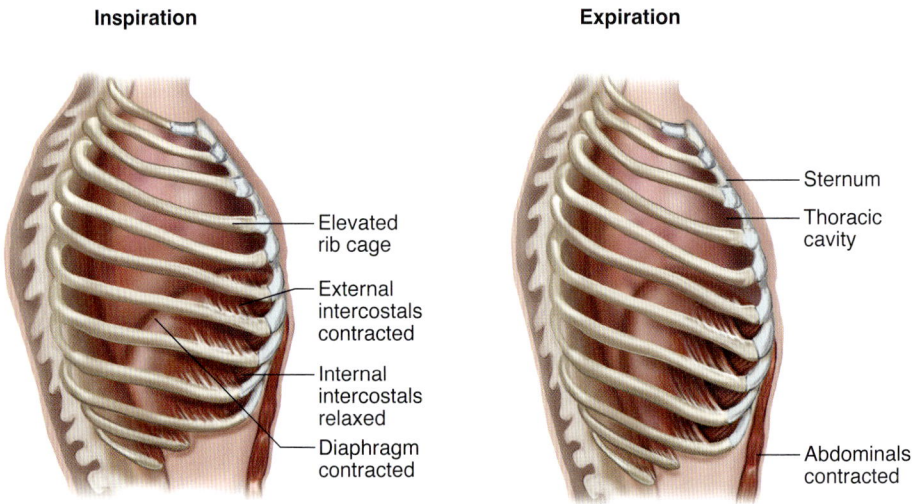

Figure 2.3 During inhalation (inspiration), the diaphragm contracts and flattens, increasing the space in the lungs and decreasing the pressure. During exhalation (expiration), the diaphragm returns to its normal shape, decreasing the space in the lungs and increasing the pressure.

influence fluid movement. Patterned breathing can help create parasympathetic responses and keep the autonomic nervous system in balance.

Other skeletal muscles can play a role in breathing based on their attachments to the ribs or sternum. Poor breathing patterns may prevent these muscles from completing their primary job in joint motion. Skeletal or other structural changes may alter the available space in the thoracic cavity. The diminished space may put stress on the associated muscles to compensate. These situations are described next.

- *Muscular influence.* Any skeletal muscle that attaches to the ribs, clavicle, or sternum has a role in breathing. When someone fails to take diaphragmatic breaths, the muscles that attach to the upper ribs and clavicle, such as the scalenes and the sternocleidomastoid, are used to pull upward on the ribs, creating more space in the thorax to allow for air exchange. Other muscles that can be used to pull up on the ribs include the pectoralis minor and the serratus anterior. In fact, one way to increase breathing capacity, such as in recovery from a sprint, is to place the hands on the knees, stabilizing the scapula and improving the ability of the accessory breathing muscles to allow for fuller rib expansion. People with breathing dysfunction, such as asthma, can benefit from treatment applied to the muscles that attach to the ribs. For specifics on treatments, see the individual muscles in chapter 3.

- *Structural influence of breathing.* Structural considerations, as outlined in chapter 4, can also influence breathing. For example, a person with lateral curvature of the spine (*scoliosis*) may have altered space in their abdominal cavity. If the abdominal organs are moved such that the diaphragm cannot flatten or the lungs cannot expand properly, breathing can become labored. Pregnancy is a natural occurrence and not a dysfunction, but it can temporarily cause similar breathing difficulties as the fetus grows and displaces the abdominal organs. The postpartum period also involves realignment of the organs as space allows, enabling the body to readjust. Therefore, for some people, breathing dysfunction and stressors put on the breathing muscles can be consistent (e.g., with scoliosis) or temporary (e.g., in pregnancy) as a result of decreased space in the abdominal cavity.

Athletes with known respiratory conditions, such as asthma, can benefit from treatment applied to the accessory breathing muscles. The muscles may become taxed in compensating for the inability of the lungs to move air properly. Typically, with asthma, the smooth muscles in the air sacs (*alveoli*) spasm and prevent proper exhalation. In turn, it takes more effort to breathe, thereby stressing breathing muscles such as the scalenes. Similar issues can be seen with respiratory illnesses that cause excessive coughing or with breathing pattern adjustments from the pain of a strained intercostal muscle. Broken or bruised ribs may also result in altered breathing patterns as a compensatory movement for pain.

For athletes, other issues beyond injuries or illness can cause respiratory muscle dysfunction. Scapular mispositioning related to scapular dyskinesis (see chapter 4) can cause the scapula to sit incorrectly on the serratus posterior superior, leading to compression and potential myofascial trigger points. Trigger points or paradoxical breathing in addition to scapular misalignment can lead to pain patterns in the serratus anterior, which can cause side-stitch pain with forced inhalation and exhalation during activity. Recognizing these potential secondary causes of breathing issues can lead to successful manual therapy treatment.

To maintain homeostasis, the body creates an environment in which more oxygen can be taken in and excess carbon dioxide can be exhaled. This environment is created by pulling the ribs up and out to give the lungs more space to take in more air. For this reason, bending over after a hard exercise effort actually decreases the space. A better response would be to place the hands in a position to stabilize the insertion of the pectoralis minor on the scapula, allowing the origin on the ribs to more fully increase the space in the thoracic cavity (see chapter 6 for more on the pectoralis minor). Recognizing poor breathing habits or patterns can help decrease myofascial pain in certain areas; it allows not only for better outcomes in aerobic capacity but also in the muscles of the extremities, because they can focus on their job in sport and not on maintaining physiological homeostasis.

Nervous System

When people think of the nervous system, they often start with the brain and spinal cord (central nervous system) as well as the peripheral nerves (peripheral nervous system). Structurally, it makes sense to start with this arrangement. Sensory information comes in from the peripheral nerves, goes to the central nervous system for a decision, and comes out via the motor nerves. Later chapters will often refer to this basic structure to help clinicians understand concepts such as the all-or-nothing principle of the motor neurons. This chapter focuses on the functional divisions of the peripheral nervous system: the somatic nervous system and, most importantly, the autonomic nervous system.

Both the somatic and autonomic nervous systems can be influenced by massage. The *somatic nervous system* relays general sensory information to the brain about what the skin, muscles, and fascia are experiencing. The *autonomic nervous system* works to create balance among the systems to keep the body in homeostasis, whether regulating breathing, heart rate, or blood pressure. A successful manual therapy treatment involves matching the desired systemic response of the body with the correct type of massage.

- *Somatic nervous system and manual therapy.* The *somatic nervous system* is responsible for controlling voluntary movement, relaying sensory information, and enabling the reflex arc. To visualize the reflex arc, imagine putting a hand on a hot stove. Because of the reflex arc, the muscles contract and the hand is pulled away before the heat sensation reaches the conscious level of the brain. General sensory information, including touch, pain, temperature, and position sensing, falls under the somatic nervous system. Therefore, the sensation of massage, including the pressure felt, is relayed by the somatic nervous system. If pressure elicits the tickle response, the somatic nervous system is responsible. If too much pressure results in pain, the somatic nervous system is again responsible. When clinicians use techniques to initiate a stretch response, this also falls under the somatic nervous system. Therefore, the somatic nervous system is an integral part of a treatment plan, and one that can be understood on a superficial level.

However, the physiological responses in connection with the autonomic nervous system are often overlooked.

The skin and fascia contain *mechanoreceptors* that respond to touch and pressure. The mechanoreceptors then change the mechanical stimuli to electrochemical activity through mechanotransduction. The sensory nerves pick up the electrochemical activity and bring it to the central nervous system for a decision on how to respond. The Pacinian corpuscles act as a receptor for quick changes in pressure as well as vibration (Schleip 2003b). As noted in the techniques outlined in chapter 3 and the additional self-care therapies described in chapter 11, percussive techniques rely on vibration, and the Pacinian corpuscles respond to these techniques to elicit change. The Ruffini organs respond to stretching of the skin and detect slow change with impulses continuing even after movement has stopped, resulting in more kinesthetic awareness to the body (Schleip 2003b). The Ruffini organ response to slower engagement of many myofascial techniques (outlined in chapter 3) not only elicits changes in the fascial system, but this response also allows that sense of change to remain for a time after treatment has ceased (Schleip 2003b). Additionally, the Ruffini organs inhibit sympathetic nervous system activity, resulting in parasympathetic dominance and the sense of relaxation that can be felt following a massage. The interplay between the treatment and the somatic nervous system, as well as the autonomic nervous system, is one of the many moving parts to an effective manual therapy treatment.

- *Autonomic nervous system.* Although it is under the control of the central nervous system, the *autonomic nervous system* is the part of the peripheral nervous system that regulates involuntary physiological processes. It is divided into the sympathetic (fight or flight) and the parasympathetic (rest and digest) components and is responsible for maintaining homeostasis of the organ systems. Despite the way these systems are often explained, a person is never truly one or the other, sympathetic or parasympathetic. The systems work together to create balance in the body, with constant fine-tuning between sympathetic and parasympathetic responses. The sympathetic nervous system prepares humans for emergencies, whereas the parasympathetic nervous system allows humans to conserve and store energy for times of emergency. The start of activity, such as exercise, requires sympathetic activity, which occurs via parasympathetic withdrawal (Robertson et al. 2004); recovery requires increased parasympathetic activity or, more specifically, sympathetic withdrawal.

When clinicians are creating a treatment plan, it is important to consider the desired effects of the manual therapy treatment on the autonomic nervous system. For example, many clinicians provide passive manual therapy treatments before the client engages in physical activity, such as before practice. However, passive treatment can engage more of the parasympathetic nervous system, which directly conflicts with the needs of a client preparing for activity (Robertson et al. 2004). Providing a more active treatment or limiting the treatment duration can better prepare the client for activity by engaging more sympathetic dominance. Relaxation massage has its purpose and would be suitable for initiating recovery after activity.

Creating a parasympathetic treatment relies on principles that encourage a return to homeostasis, including decreased blood pressure and heart rate and increased heart rate variability and gastric mobility (Cambron et al. 2006; Resnick 2016). Slower techniques should be considered, such as *myofascial glides*, which engage the myofascial tissue at a slow pace, or *effleurage*, which comprises a gliding stroke often used to introduce the massage or to spread emollient. Techniques such as *petrissage* (a kneading technique involving lifting and squeezing the tissue) can be performed at a slower pace. Movement techniques can be passive rather than active. The treatment duration can be longer (e.g., >20 minutes), and the amount of movement to change position should be limited. The amount of pressure used should be tolerable, not eliciting a response of either pain or ticklishness. In addition, the environment should promote relaxation and comfort. These treatments are often reserved for use after activity or on recovery days, because parasympathetic dominance before activity or competition is not preferred.

When sympathetic dominance is required, such as before activity or competition, the treatment must have an opposing approach. The treatment duration should be shorter; however, no specific parameters have been investigated because most of the research focuses on one area, recommending a duration of up to 12 minutes (Poppendieck et al. 2016). Techniques should be performed at a quicker pace, which is more stimulating to the sympathetic nervous system. Movement can allow for more active engagement by the participant, and pressure, although still under a painful stimulus, can be more stimulating. In addition, to prevent the client from getting too comfortable, position changes can be more frequent in this setting compared with a relaxing treatment. The client should emerge from this type of treatment more stimulated than relaxed as well as prepared and ready to engage in physical activity.

Effect of Manual Therapy on the Cardiovascular, Myofascial, and Nervous Systems

The intersection between the cardiovascular and nervous systems can initiate many of the physiological changes that occur with manual therapy. It is not just the pressure of massage that can influence fluid movement in the cardiovascular system; the autonomic nervous system response to alter fluid dynamics and the pressure response to relax the muscles can also bring about fluid movement. The somatic nervous system response brings about change through eliciting the mechanoreceptors to soften the structures, allowing for better fluid movement. What makes the treatment most effective is the clinician's understanding of how all the systems interconnect to create the desired results. However, the lack of such understanding can lead to a mismatch between patient goals and treatment outcomes. This section will attempt to clarify some of the processes working together to create a physiologically balanced manual therapy treatment.

When the goals of a manual therapy treatment are to increase blood flow to the area, in addition to changes in pressure and increased histamine release, withdrawal of resting sympathetic tone (meaning parasympathetic activity will be greater) results in vasodilation to the local blood vessels. The sympathetic nervous system typically elicits vasoconstriction—which is important as eliciting contraction of the smooth muscles of the veins can help guide the fluid in the venous system back to the heart. Although vasoconstriction occurs from sympathetic dominance and vasodilation occurs from parasympathetic dominance, mechanisms are in place to balance the two. For example, the pathways responsible for vasodilation in the muscles and skin are independent. Therefore, if a more superficial technique is used, such as to initiate a response of the lymphatic system or superficial venous system close to the skin surface, vasoconstriction can occur while vasodilation can be initiated in the muscles. With increased metabolic activity, autoregulation of blood flow results (i.e., a greater need for energy increases blood flow). Increased metabolic activity supersedes the sympathetic response of vasoconstriction, such as with exercise in which the arterioles of the working muscles vasodilate to compensate for the need for more energy. Therefore, even a treatment that intends to provide more sympathetic dominance can still allow for increased blood flow to the area as needed.

All the changes in the circulatory and autonomic nervous systems positively affect muscle physiology. Muscle contraction requires energy, as outlined in chapter 1 (see the discussion of sliding filament theory). At the same time, ending a muscle contraction also requires energy. When there is not enough energy around the open binding sites, calcium cannot flow back into the sarcoplasmic reticulum. With calcium still present, the binding sites remain open, and the contraction is sustained owing to lack of energy (see the discussion of trigger points in chapter 3). By increasing blood flow to the area being treated, relaxation of the muscle is introduced through stopping a sustained contraction. As demonstrated in later chapters, the presence of trigger points will weaken the muscle. The ability to increase blood flow into the area can correct deficiencies in the muscles.

WHY DOES THE CLINICIAN CARE?

To relieve tension in the muscles, clinicians want to work with the circulatory systems, respiratory system, and autonomic nervous system and apply their knowledge of muscle physiology and fascia to create the desired change. Chapter 3 introduces the intent of the manual therapy techniques. To create a balanced approach, clinicians need to select the correct technique for the correct system they are looking to influence. Chapters 6 to 10 in part II describe the specific muscles and some of the biomechanical stressors. Along the way, clinicians will continue to keep in mind the goals of the patient, along with the best evidence and the best approach to treatment. When creating the best treatment plan, clinicians also must always consider the treatment intent and how the body responds.

Types of Manual Therapies

Not all manual therapies are created the same. It is important for clinicians to use the correct type of technique depending on the tissue and the condition. Many introductory massage classes for athletic trainers and physical therapists introduce effleurage, petrissage, and tapotement (percussion), which are discussed in detail later in this chapter. Massage therapists learn these techniques as part of Swedish massage, which is more of a circulatory treatment. Although these are effective strokes, they may not be appropriate in all clinical settings or for all conditions. For example, a massage therapist may use creams or lotions, which are not allowed in some sports (e.g., wrestling) or may cause inadequate heat dissipation for someone participating in an outdoor sport, increasing the chance of heat illness. In some cases, the treatment given does not correspond with the physiological response wanted, as outlined in chapter 2. Therefore, it is important for clinicians to know both how the body systems respond and the treatments that correspond with the desired response.

Intent is a large part of effective manual therapy. When the treatment matches the intent, the results seem like magic.

Circulatory Treatments

Circulatory treatments affect circulation in the body, including the cardiovascular and lymphatic systems. The purpose of this type of massage is to influence the movement of fluid through the vessels. In relation to the cardiovascular system, massage encourages blood flow to and from the tissues. To influence the arterial aspect, the techniques used must have enough compression to release deeper structures or should use muscle movement to encourage blood flow into the area. The muscle movement can be active or passive, depending on the treatment intent. To influence venous flow, more strokes gliding proximally to distally would be used. To influence the lymphatic system, the pressure applied is usually very light, and the strokes used present more of a drag with slower movements. Lymphatic drainage massage is not in the scope of this text, but the understanding of the role of the lymphatic treatment is. While all massage has some influence on the circulatory systems, it is important for clinicians to understand the intent of the treatment and apply appropriate techniques to create the desired response.

Common types of circulatory massage include relaxation massage, lymphatic techniques, and intermittent compression. Each is described next.

- *Relaxation massage.* The term *Swedish massage* is typically synonymous with *relaxation massage*. The clinician usually uses strokes that are a bit more superficial, applied with an emollient. Although this is a therapeutic treatment, typically the emphasis is more on relaxation and less on a specific ailment. Physiologically, relaxation massage results in increased local circulation, decreased blood pressure, and increased parasympathetic activity (Cambron et al. 2006; Resnick 2016). The strokes associated with this type of massage include, but are not limited to, effleurage, petrissage, and percussion. These strokes are explained in more detail in the Massage Techniques section of this chapter.

- *Lymphatic techniques.* Techniques for treatment of the lymphatic system include lymphatic drainage and lymphatic facilitation, which are taught in depth by other entities. Because specialized training is needed for this type of treatment, lymphatic techniques will not be explained in depth here. For athletes, lymphatic facilitation by a trained practitioner can be used for acute inflammation. Without distinct training, the clinician may push fluid into the lymphatic system, which can lead to secondary problems. For example, overloading the lymphatic system can lead to feelings of listlessness or fatigue. Many untrained practitioners think they are using techniques to influence inflammation removal; however, they often use too much pressure for the delicate lymphatic vessels.

- *Intermittent compression.* This type of compression can be used to facilitate fluid movement through the circulatory system by changing the pressures in the vessels. This technique can be performed with manual compression (as listed in the Massage Techniques section later in this chapter) or with intermittent compression modalities (discussed more in chapter 11).

Myofascial Treatments

Myofascial treatments work within the myofascial unit. The principles of muscles and fascia outlined in chapter 1 create the building blocks for myofascial treatments. These treatments typically do not use an emollient, and they involve very slow engagement with the tissues. Change in fascia occurs slowly, whether it be from the stressors put on the fascia from everyday activities, including sports, or from the application of manual therapy to the tissues.

Myofascial Release

Myofascial release refers to any technique used to alter the fascia or relieve myofascial pain. Myofascial release can take a variety of forms, from myofascial glides to skin rolling to active release techniques. These techniques are outlined next, and they are designed to work with the nuances of the myofascial system.

- *Myofascial compression* involves using techniques that push down into the fascia. Examples include instrument-assisted soft tissue mobilization or even foam rolling. These techniques compress the fascia and attempt to alter tensegrity properties. Foam rolling and other self-care techniques are outlined in chapter 11. Instrument-assisted techniques are outside the scope of this text but will be offered as a solution in chapters 6 to 10 for clinicians with the appropriate training.

- *Myofascial decompression* is a technique that lifts the fascia, creating space underneath the skin surface. Decompression allows for fluid movement into the area. Cupping is one of the most common techniques for myofascial decompression: Air is sucked out of the cups, creating a vacuum that pulls up the skin. After a cupping treatment, it is normal to experience darkened spots where the blood pooled under the skin surface. Decompression can be combined with movement, in which the cups are placed in areas and the body part is brought through various ranges of motion. The exact decompression technique will not be discussed in this book; however, it may be pointed out as a potential treatment choice in chapters 6 to 10.

Fascial Layers and Massage Treatment

The *superficial fascia* is a fibrous layer of loosely packed collagen and abundant elastic fibers (Stecco et al. 2016). The lymphatic vessels and superficial veins are contained in this fascial layer. Treatment for the superficial fascia includes more superficial massage strokes targeting a broader area. Massage strokes such as effleurage are effective on venous return, provided they are broader and more superficial in nature. Strokes that are more effective on the lymphatic vessels provide only enough pressure to elicit a dermal stretch.

The *deep fascia*—the dense, fibrous layers and the epimysial layer over the muscles—respond to more targeted manipulation with a smaller surface area (Stecco et al. 2016). Myofascial treatments for these areas can be broad, addressing the entire fascial structure, including those outside the areas of concern. Additionally, when an area of restriction is identified, a more specific and concentrated approach can be taken.

There are two considerations to keep in mind about manual therapy and pressure: Providing work to the deep fascia does not necessarily coincide with using more pressure down into the structures, nor does pushing fluid through the venous and lymphatic systems require increased pressure to move the fluid. Too much pressure can have negative consequences. The amount of pressure needed to enhance venous flow actually closes the lymphatic capillaries, preventing uptake of the lymphatic fluid. In addition, the amount of pressure to create manipulation in the deep myofascial layers could be too much to optimize fluid movement. It is also important to note the thixotropic nature of fascia, allowing it to move from a gel state to a sol state. Slow, sustained pressure will allow for deformation of the fascia, while quick, hard pressure will lead to resistance. Forcing the fascia will have the opposite effect because the tension will build.

Muscle Tissue and Massage Treatment

The properties of muscle as outlined in chapter 1 are part of the building blocks of a manual therapy treatment. Regarding pressure, muscles respond to mechanical stimuli (*excitability*) and develop tension when stimulated (*contractility*). Therefore, consistently providing too much pressure can potentially cause contraction, instead of relaxation, of the muscle. Muscles also are *extensible*, meaning that clinicians can provide passive stretching during the treatment without permanent deformation to muscles, and *elastic*, meaning muscles will return to their original shape following treatment. These properties can be used to enhance the treatment by allowing the clinician to incorporate movement in a variety of techniques. Some myofascial techniques outlined later in this chapter (e.g., pin and stretch) can be used to assist in gaining range of motion in the muscles.

Muscles under stress can be subject to a variety of dysfunctions, from knots or tender points to trigger points. These dysfunctions can prevent the muscle fibers or motor units from producing an effective contraction, thereby limiting the muscle's ability to do its job.

- *Trigger points* are hyperirritable nodules within a muscle that cause pain and elicit a predicted referral pattern when compressed. Although most trigger point referrals are pain in a distal part of the body, active trigger points can lead to other symptoms, including headache, nausea, and dizziness. The area of the trigger point gives a local twitch response, and treatment may result in soreness.

The cause of trigger points relies on theories well documented by Travell and Simons (1983). A commonly accepted theory suggests that a sustained release of calcium creates sustained shortening of the sarcomeres; when calcium is present, the binding sites remain open, and the contraction is sustained. When the area is contracted, it is not available for recruitment by the motor unit for a subsequent contraction. The contraction, however, remains in a more localized area of the sarcomere, not necessarily the full muscle fiber. Returning to an earlier example in chapter 1, if the contraction to lift a set amount of weight requires the recruitment of 200 motor units and only 190 are available because of a trigger point, the muscle will not be at full strength. Although this example is an oversimplification for illustrative purposes, the reasoning remains that a muscle with trigger points is potentially inefficient in doing its job. Additionally, the trigger point may cause referred pain, which could be mistaken as a different injury.

- *Tender points* are areas of tenderness in a muscle that do not meet the definition of a trigger point, meaning there is neither a predicted pain referral pattern nor an elicited twitch response. Tender points are sometimes referred to as *knots*, although no source gives a specific definition for the lay term.

To describe a knot, I tend to use the spaghetti analogy. When spaghetti is drained after cooking, the spaghetti strands clump together if left alone. To prevent clumping, either rinse the starch off the spaghetti or add a liquid, such as sauce or olive oil. Following this thought process, the muscle fibers become matted and clump together because of a lack of fluid movement (blood, interstitial fluid, plasma, etc.), and the fascia binds down and adheres to the area. Massage is used to increase fluid into the area, which separates the clumps or even prevents them from forming, like the liquid introduced to drained spaghetti.

Using Muscle and Fascia Physiology for Effective Outcomes

The information about muscle and fascia learned in chapter 1 can also be applied to some of the physiology laws discussed previously, which are effective in manual therapy techniques. For example, postisometric relaxation and reciprocal inhibition relax the muscle and can be incorporated in a treatment. Whether clinicians choose to use only contraction with stretching to gain range of motion or contraction in combination with the massage techniques outlined next, they can create an effective treatment to affect range of motion. Physiology laws can be integrated into treatment to create balance in the muscles as needed. Keep in mind when working with athletes that not all postural distortions can be fixed. Some posture variations are necessary for sport performance. The clinician's goal is not to fix what is not broken but rather to relieve tension in the muscles, allow for proper muscle contraction and alignment, and reduce fatigue. All of these benefits of massage will aid in injury prevention, performance, and recovery.

This section revisits the discussion in chapter 1 on postural and phasic muscles and puts it in the context of building a manual therapy treatment. Recall the previous discussion of the pectoralis minor (postural muscle, scapular protractor) and the rhomboids (phasic muscles, scapular retractors): Clinicians need to consider how each muscle will respond to stress and which treatments would work best. Many people with upper back pain centered between the scapulae will feel like they need to stretch this area. However, because phasic rhomboids respond to stress by lengthening, stretching is the wrong choice of treatment because it would further lengthen the muscles. The postural pectoralis minor, which is shortened in response to stress, would not only benefit from stretching, but also the stretching of the postural muscle would relieve that feeling of needing to be stretched from the rhomboids. Stretching the scapular protractors eases tension on the scapular retractors, muscles that are trying to hang on to the medial border of the scapula as it is being pulled away.

Massage Techniques

This section will discuss a variety of common massage techniques. Although many of these techniques fall under the categories described earlier (e.g., circulatory or myofascial), they are discussed here to highlight how they can be used separately and together to create a sports massage protocol.

When performing massage, body mechanics is of utmost importance (figure 3.1). Relying too much on just the thumbs or hands without using different tools or body weight to assist can result in injury to the clinician performing the treatment, especially when the clinician provides multiple treatments per day (Resnick 2024). General body mechanics for clinicians includes the following rules:

- Maintain a split stance: Your legs should be in a lunge position when you are alongside the table (figure 3.1*a*) and in a squat position when you are facing the table (figure 3.1*b*).
- Movement should be from your torso where the legs and hips move your upper body.

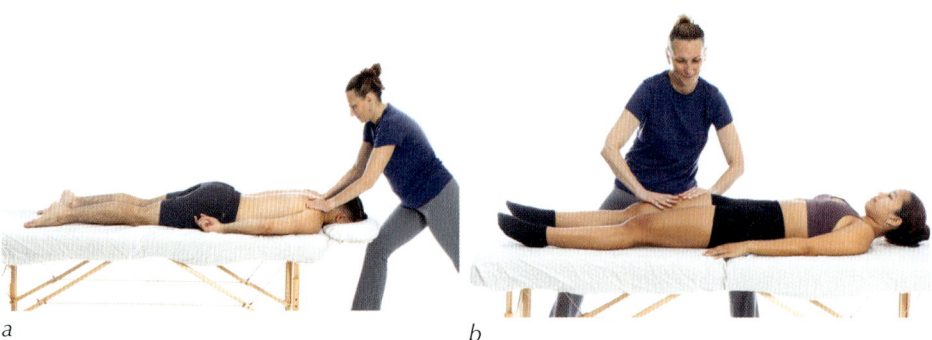

Figure 3.1 Lunge, split stance position with the back straight and the head forward. (b) Squat position facing the table with the legs wide, knees soft, and back straight.

- Keep your back straight, avoiding excessive flexion.
- Adjust the table height as necessary to fit your own mechanics and the size of the client on the table (including if moving the client to a side-lying position).
- Keep your wrists in a neutral position, avoiding hyperextension.

The treatment area for massage should allow for appropriate body mechanics. There should be enough room for the clinician to move around the massage table. Otherwise, the patient's position should be adjusted for optimal reach. Because many techniques of sports massage are performed in an open clinic, the patient will typically be clothed; this is different from a traditional massage setting in which draping provides boundaries. By working around and over clothing, it is easier to change position with the patient on the table and to use movement in many of the techniques. (*Note:* Clothing is a boundary that should be respected, with the clinician working over clothing and never under clothing.)

Common Swedish Massage Techniques

Some common techniques typically fall under the category of Swedish massage; however, a few can be done in other types of treatment. Hallmarks of Swedish massage include the use of oils or lotions, the emphasis on circulatory system influences, and the promotion of relaxation. Some techniques, such as percussion and petrissage, can be done in conjunction with multiple types of treatments. Other techniques that I consider to be more of a crossover or a cousin to a technique, such as effleurage in Swedish massage and glides in myofascial treatment, can also be used.

EFFLEURAGE

Effleurage is a gliding stroke that is often used to introduce touch at the start of massage, to transition between strokes or body parts, and to apply any lubricant to the area (figure 3.2). Although effleurage is typically a superficial application, pressure, speed, and drag can be altered based on the intent of the session. When

Chapter 3 Types of Manual Therapies 35

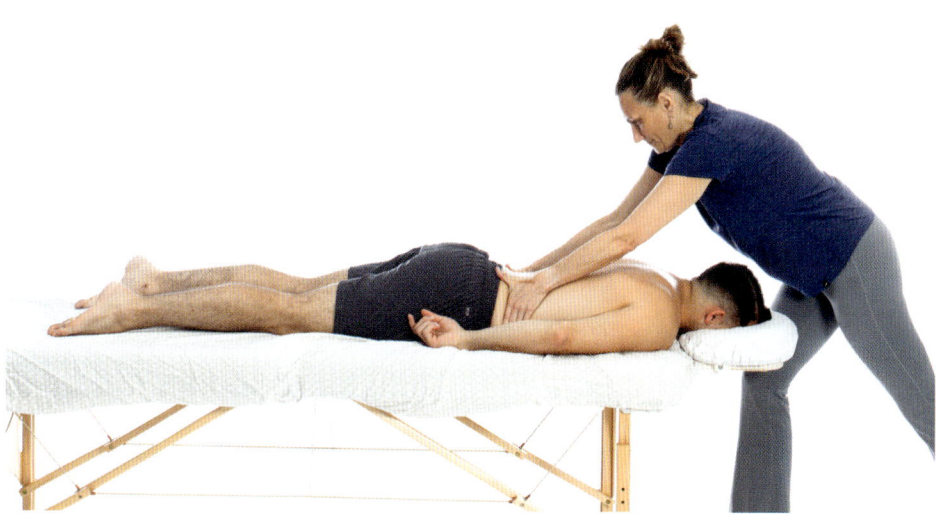

Figure 3.2 Effleurage performed on the back has the hands making full contact on the skin and the hips and legs driving the arm movement.

the effleurage is more superficial and slower, it can be soothing and promote parasympathetic activity. An effleurage with more pressure at a slow rate can also elicit a parasympathetic response. However, whether the effleurage is superficial or deep, the body responds with a more sympathetic response when a faster rate is used. Although effleurage is usually part of a Swedish massage and is used to promote parasympathetic dominance, a quicker-paced effleurage can be used in instances where more a sympathetic response is desired. In addition, clinicians should use caution in situations where emollient is not wanted; examples include for a wrestler before competition when it may be against the rules or for any athlete competing in an outdoor climate where they may have difficulty dissipating heat with lubricant on the skin.

Effleurage uses your entire hand, from palms to fingertips, with the pressure equally distributed throughout the hand. Your wrists should remain as neutral as possible (avoid hyperextension of the wrist). Pressure should not come from your hands or shoulders but from the weight of the body behind the hands.

PETRISSAGE

Petrissage is a kneading technique that uses alternating and squeezing to lift the tissue, typically focusing on the muscle belly (figure 3.3). When the muscle belly is squeezed, the muscle spindles are activated and lifting of the muscle puts a stretch on the tendon, activating the Golgi tendon organs. The result is relaxation of the muscles. Compression and heat of the hands on the tissue leads to a softening of the fascial layers, starting with the superficial fascia. Like with effleurage, the pace of the petrissage influences the intent. A slower petrissage will create a more parasympathetic state, whereas a quicker pace with a deeper grasp of the tissue will have a more sympathetic influence. Petrissage can be done with or without emollient and also over clothing.

To execute the petrissage technique, your full hand and fingers should be in contact with and compress the tissue while you move along the muscle belly. Squeezing should occur from your palms to fingertips (think of squeezing toothpaste down the length of a tube, rather than compressing a plastic water bottle). Combine the squeezing with a lifting of the tissue. When performing petrissage, your body should face the table, your legs should be in a plié squat position, and your hips should rock back and forth in time with your hands to create the rhythm of the movement.

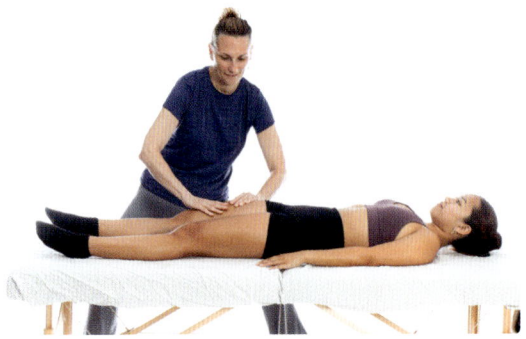

Figure 3.3 Petrissage uses the full hands to alternate compressing the tissue then picking up and squeezing from the palms to the fingertips as the lower body moves from side to side.

JOSTLING OR SHAKING

Jostling or *shaking* is a vigorous movement of the tissue (figure 3.4). You can pick up the tissue from the bone (e.g., the quadriceps), shake the limb (e.g., the arm), or move the muscles from side to side (e.g., the erector spinae group of the spine). The technique should be performed as a rhythmic movement of the tissues, with the intent of stimulating the mechanoreceptors. When the full limb is involved, the mechanoreceptors in the joint capsule are also stimulated. Before you perform this technique, it is important to know whether the client has a history of instability in the joint, especially the glenohumeral joint.

Mechanics for the jostling or shaking technique involve you utilizing the lunge stance of your legs. Your full hand should be used to pick up the tissue. This technique is intended to be done at a quick pace, meaning it will have more of a sympathetic influence. Like all techniques, jostling or shaking takes practice; it may feel awkward to you until you have mastered it.

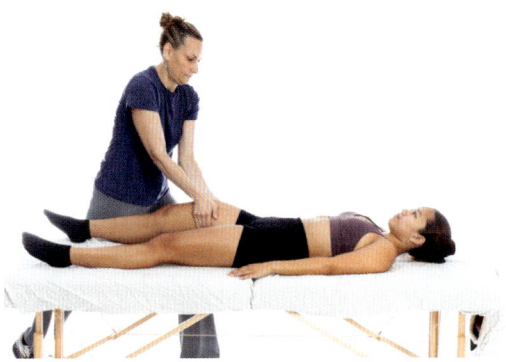

Figure 3.4 Jostling of the leg involves starting proximally by picking up the quadriceps muscle and quickly putting it down; work your way down the leg toward the feet in an alternating rhythm.

FRICTION

Friction is used to move the tissue underneath the skin and can be applied transversely or parallel to the fibers (figure 3.5). Superficial friction done quickly and with little pressure can be used to warm the area. With increased pressure, friction will both compress and stretch the tissues. Friction is another technique that can be done with or without emollient, keeping in mind that the stretch is enhanced without emollient because it is easier to engage with the tissue. Although friction can be used as a general technique over an area, most people associate friction with *cross-fiber friction*, which is a more specific technique used to address a specific area. Cross-fiber friction is effective for specific areas, such as with postoperative surgical scars, but may be too specific for many of the sports massage scenarios presented here.

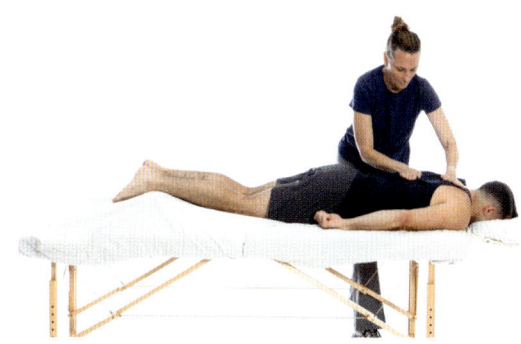

Figure 3.5 Friction can be performed over clothing with a full hand moving around the tissue quickly with little pressure.

COMPRESSION

Compression involves pushing down into the tissue with varying force, followed by release of the tissue (figure 3.6). Pushing into the muscle and the subsequent release can stimulate the release of histamine, keep blood flowing in the muscles, and stretch the muscle. This technique does not use emollient and thus is a good way to warm up the tissue before a sports massage treatment that does not rely on any lubricant. Compression can be used similar to effleurage in examining and preparing the tissue for treatment; however, unlike effleurage, compression can be done over clothing. Compression also creates more of a sympathetic response, making it appropriate to prepare the body for activity.

The most ideal hand position for applying compression uses a loose fist. This position is preferred because it allows you to maintain a neutral wrist. It is also less invasive because open hands and flat palms should be avoided on areas such as the gluteal region, where compression is an effective technique. You should use the split stance or lunge technique when positioned alongside the table, or you should use a squat stance if you are facing the table.

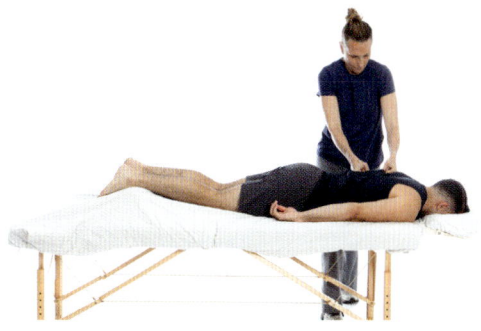

Figure 3.6 A loose fist is used to compress the tissues on the back over clothing; pronation and supination of the forearm are used to create a twisting motion.

PERCUSSION (OR TAPOTEMENT OR VIBRATION)

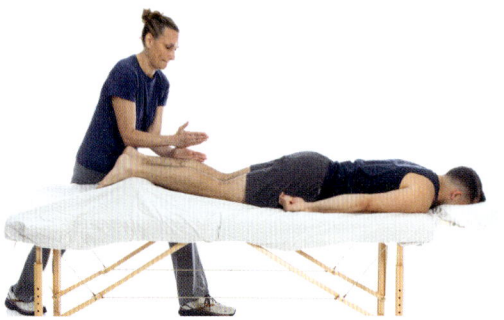

Figure 3.7 Hacking using the ulnar border of an open hand is done parallel to the muscle fibers of the gastrocnemius.

Percussion, also referred to as *tapotement* or *vibration*, involves application of mechanical vibration to the myofascial system (figure 3.7). Percussion is purported to influence the stretch receptors in the muscles, creating relaxation using similar mechanisms to reciprocal inhibition. In addition to reducing muscle tension, the vibratory effect also alters fascial mobility via changes in viscoelasticity. The vibration also causes the release of histamine, which is noted by the red color of the skin over the area of application and may allow for greater pain tolerance. Percussive techniques increase blood flow to the area, possibly because of muscle contraction and relaxation allowing for greater blood perfusion (Ferreira et al. 2023).

The application of percussive techniques in manual therapy includes the following:

- *Hacking* involves using the ulnar border (pinky side) of an open hand. Hacking should be done parallel to the muscle fibers.
- *Beating* or *drumming* involves using the ulnar side of a loose fist.
- *Cupping* involves using a cupped palm of the hand, with the borders of the hand used to make contact.

Changing the speed, tempo, and force of the movement will alter the body's response.

Myofascial Techniques

Myofascial techniques are designed to engage the myofascial system. As discussed in chapter 1, fascia surrounds the entire body, so the techniques described next may be more general. However, once clinicians understand the basic types of techniques, they can adjust them to the specific muscle properties in creating a treatment. The specifics of how to apply myofascial techniques to the muscles are outlined in chapters 6 to 10.

SPIRALING

Spiraling engages some of the relevant fascia structures surrounding the thigh, the upper arm, and the torso as well as the fascial layers below (figure 3.8). It is important to note that spiraling is done only in areas where the muscles form more of a cylinder (e.g., muscles of the abdomen and low back) or those surrounding a bone (e.g., muscles of the thigh). Spiraling cannot be done on the lower leg or the forearm where the muscles are attached between the two bones. The technique is a good way to initiate warming and mobilizing the fascia surrounding the body part prior to further treatment.

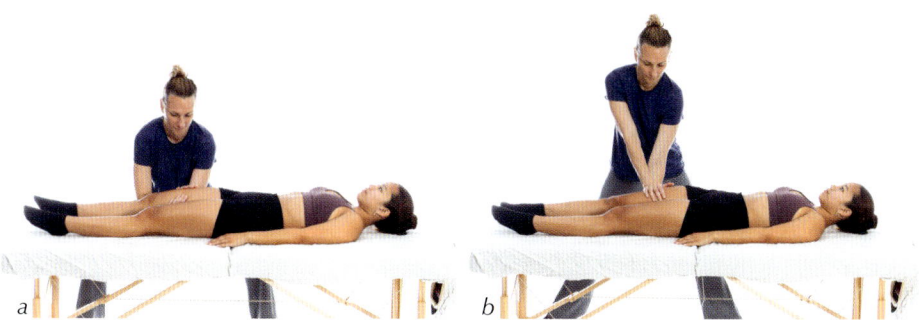

Figure 3.8 *(a)* The start of the spiral where the underneath hand reaches all the way around to the medial thigh and the top hand is lateral; the therapist is in a deep squat. *(b)* The ending position where the underneath hand is drawn lateral and the top hand pushes the tissue medial; the therapist has "stood up."

For the leg and torso, spiraling is performed with the patient lying supine and you facing the table in a squat stance. Reach one hand under the area as far as possible (e.g., the most medial and anterior aspect of the thigh) and start the other hand closer to your body (e.g., on the posterior lateral aspect of the thigh). To initiate the spiral, stand up out of the squat while your bottom hand pulls the tissue more laterally and your top hand pushes the tissue medially, spiraling the tissue. The push and pull creates a unique fascial stretch to the area.

MYOFASCIAL GLIDES

As noted earlier, myofascial glides are similar to effleurage, but no emollient is used on the skin and the goal is to engage with the fascia. One difference between the two techniques is that myofascial glides are meant to be slow, with you allowing the melting or release of the fascia to guide your hand, as opposed to using your hand to guide the movement over the skin as done with effleurage. The stance is similar: Use a split-lunge stance to the side of the table and move your torso as the hand glides. The entire heel of your hand, a loose fist using the proximal phalanges, or even the forearm can be used to provide the glide. When you are using the forearm, your legs will need to drop to a lower lunge, but the advantage is the forearm is able to cover more surface area of the body. The key to an effective glide is patience. See chapter 7 (trapezius section) or chapter 8 (low back section) for examples of glides.

SKIN ROLLING

Skin rolling involves lifting the skin to warm and release the superficial fascia (figure 3.9). Skin rolling is a form of petrissage, which is not as deep because it does not pick up the muscle. For those who may be familiar, the technique is similar to picking up the skin to measure a skin fold during a body fat assessment. Grasp the tissue between the thumb and the rest of the fingers. Your thumb guides the roll; like the myofascial glides, the roll should not be forced. Your body should be positioned appropriately in the direction of the roll, which is dependent on the direction of the fascia.

There are several situations in which skin rolling can be difficult to perform. When the client is not well hydrated, the superficial layer will adhere to the structures below. It will also be difficult to lift the skin if there are adhesions. Skin rolling might be more difficult after an endurance event or maximal lift. When the muscles are energy depleted, often the fascia can be adhered. Depending on the sport or the patient's stressors, certain areas of the body may be difficult to roll. Also, of all the techniques listed, skin rolling has the most variability among patients. Some people just do not like this technique; therefore, it should be avoided based on patient preferences. Other techniques can be used to elicit the same response.

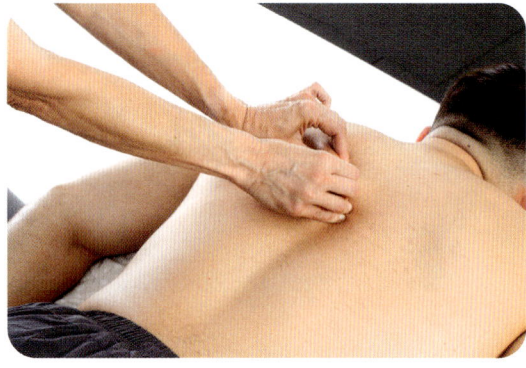

Figure 3.9 In the skin rolling technique, the fascia of the upper back, superficial to the trapezius muscle, is grasped between the thumb and the rest of the fingers. The direction of the treatment here is angled toward the head following the fascial lines.

LIFT AND SHIFT

Lift and shift combines petrissage (lifting the muscle) with compression and stretch. In this technique, the entire muscle is grasped between the thumb and fingers. From there, it can be lifted or shifted, pulling away from the origin or insertion. For example, the latissimus dorsi can be grasped and then distracted from the origin at the ribs and thoracolumbar fascia or from the humerus (see chapter 6, figure 6.17*b*). Additionally, movement can be added where the latissimus dorsi is distracted from the humerus while the patient attempts to bring their hand above their head into flexion. This technique creates a stretch in the muscle and can be used effectively for postural muscles.

PIN AND STRETCH

Pin and stretch is a type of compression that can add either passive or active movement. The technique is performed by shortening the muscle passively (performing the action), holding a spot on the muscle or tendon, and then slowly lengthening the muscle (performing the opposite motion of the muscle's action). When the muscle is passively lengthening, it allows for a unique stretch to the area between the spot of the pin and the insertion of the muscle. The pin and stretch can be done multiple times from the insertion toward the origin of the muscle. Ideally, no emollient should be used with this technique because it allows for deeper engagement of the tissue. Specific examples of how to perform the pin and stretch will be addressed in the individual muscle chapters; for an example of the pin and stretch of the hamstrings, see chapter 9, figure 9.8*a-b*.

If the technique is adjusted to passively pin and have the patient actively contract the antagonist, it becomes more of an active technique. Because fascia and muscle like movement, the patient may feel even more of a stretch. The pin and stretch is also an example of reciprocal inhibition (contraction of the antagonist), allowing for a greater stretch of the agonist. This technique can also be applied using a myofascial glide during the stretch. The patient actively goes through the range of motion while you glide proximally. This technique adds an additional element of gliding during the active movement. The order of application would be to start passively, then change to active movement, and then use active movement with a glide.

Massage Contraindications

There are some basic contraindications for massage that all manual therapy practitioners need to consider, although the following discussion is not exhaustive. Contraindications can be *systemic*, meaning no massage should be performed at all, or they can be *local*, meaning massage is acceptable but the area of concern should be avoided. Systemic contraindications include fever and edema of unknown origin. Local contraindications include open wounds, skin infections, and varicose veins. Although cancer is not a contraindication, clinicians should not perform manual therapy without proper training in massage for patients undergoing cancer treatment. Patients with cancer may have areas of skin sensitivity or contraindications based on their treatment regimen. Pregnancy is not a contraindication for massage; however, proper training is needed for correct positioning of a pregnant patient, and some range-of-motion techniques should be avoided because the hormone relaxin is released in later stages of pregnancy. For more comprehensive lists of contraindications, clinicians should consult a pathology reference.

Emollients

When talking about massage, many people assume all treatments start with some sort of emollient or lubricant applied to the skin. However, the purpose of these substances is to reduce the drag on the skin. The more lubricant used or the more liquid the lubricant, the less drag. When performing treatments such as myofascial release in which engagement in the tissue is necessary for an effective treatment, use of any lubricant can prevent engagement. Use of too much lubricant can lead to gliding over the skin, which is not the goal of a therapeutic treatment. For a client with excessive body hair in an area, the use of a minimal amount of lubricant may be desired to make gliding strokes more comfortable.

Some emollients, such as oil or lotion, are considered high drag and prevent effective tissue engagement, especially if large amounts are used. These emollients may also leave a greasy feeling on the skin. Other emollients, such as creams or salves, may be preferred to provide low amounts of drag, still allowing for engagement in the tissues but making the treatment more comfortable for the patient on the table. Working with athletes, however, brings the added concern of using any emollient before competition. As noted earlier, in some sports (e.g., wrestling), using any lubricant on the skin may not be allowed prior to competition. For endurance events (e.g., a marathon or distance triathlon) or any activity in warm weather, lubricants on the skin may prevent heat dissipation, leaving the person more vulnerable to heat illness. For these reasons, avoiding lubricant use is preferred prior to an event. If any emollient is used, it is important to remove as much as possible following the treatment.

WHY DOES THE CLINICIAN CARE?

When clinicians build treatments around the stresses of the muscle, sometimes they need to change their style of thinking. Of course, the goals of patients are important, but so is educating them about their body and how the body responds to the stresses put on it.

Manual therapy treatment, especially in clients with chronic conditions, involves a balance of attending to the areas of complaint along with treating the areas causing the complaint. Thus, practitioners cannot cure the issue in one treatment. Chapter 4, on structural and functional considerations related to sport, will describe how these issues result in the stresses put on the body. For some sports, practitioners can relieve the discomfort and work with the dysfunction, but they must keep in mind that the continued stress of training will continue to lead to dysfunction—and that is okay. They need to then work within these parameters.

It is also important to match the manual therapy treatment with the correct physiological response. One common example is when a client asks for a "flush" massage to decrease delayed-onset muscle soreness. In providing this massage, many times the practitioner will use a lot of pressure, either because that is what they were taught or because that is what the patient requested. However, using a lot of pressure does not best influence either the lymphatic system or the venous return, both of which require a lighter touch. Although this type of massage might feel good and might relieve soreness, it is a mismatch between the intent of the treatment and the goals of the session.

Structural Versus Functional Considerations

When examining the body, it is important for clinicians to differentiate between issues that might be structural or functional. Structural issues involve the skeleton and joint structures. Functional issues involve the muscles and fascia. Identifying where issues originate is an important consideration when developing a manual therapy treatment.

Structural Issues

Structural considerations are based on the bones, ligaments, and cartilage (figure 4.1). Examples of structural issues include (but are not limited to) labral tears, meniscal tears, limb length, and disc pathology. Structural issues cannot be changed through manual therapy. However, clinicians can work with associated soft tissue structures to relieve tension and improve range of motion.

Some structural issues can be repaired surgically, and manual therapy can be used before surgery to relieve symptoms or after surgery to assist in the recovery process. After surgery, it is important to always follow physician advice until the client is cleared for a particular activity (range of motion, walking, etc.) before initiating any massage treatment. Surgery may fix the problem but the body may never return to its previously healthy state, continuing to rely on poor habits or creating new pathways that may be inefficient. If the structure cannot be fixed, the body can adapt; however, adaptation could lead to ineffective or insufficient muscle firing patterns. Mechanics may be compromised, and muscles may fatigue more quickly. It is important for both clinicians and patients to understand that changes with manual therapy are not permanent and will require frequent attention. Patient education on this topic is very important, because patients may expect miracles.

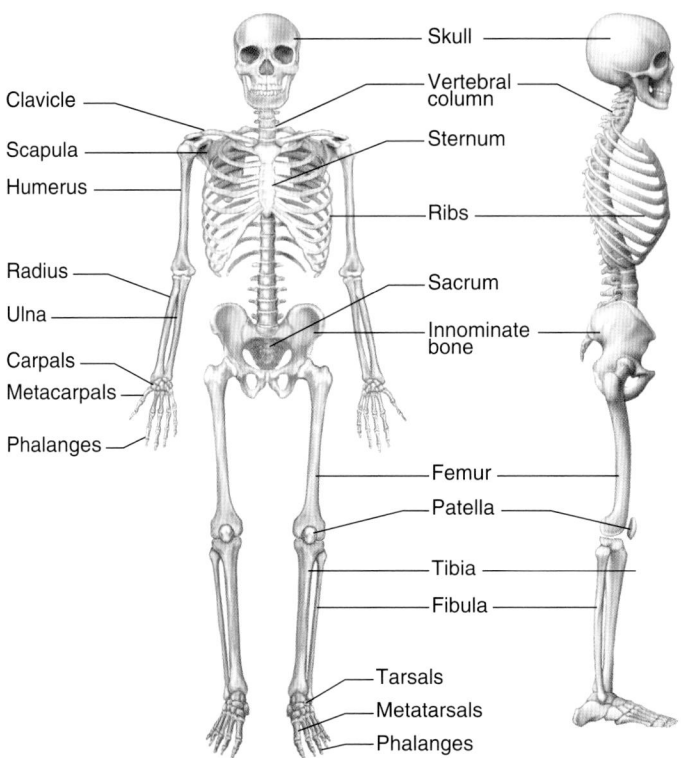

Figure 4.1 The skeleton is the framework of the body. While injuries to bones, ligaments, and cartilage cannot be fixed with manual therapy, the compensatory deficiencies in the muscle can be relieved, if only temporarily.

Examples of Common Structural Problems and Considerations of the Bone Structure

This section will discuss some common problems in the bone structure and how manual therapy can be used effectively to relieve symptoms. Bone issues are not just linked to fractures and postfracture healing. Examples of common structural problems include a structural leg-length issue, spinal misalignment (e.g., scoliosis), unequal bone size (e.g., small hemipelvis), or bone spurs in tendons (e.g., leading to chronic tendinosis), among others.

SCOLIOSIS

Scoliosis is a lateral curvature of the spine. This condition can create either a C-shaped curve or an S-shaped curve within the vertebrae. Scoliosis can be related to functional concerns, in which unilateral shortening of the quadratus lumborum can lead to a spinal curve (see the Lateral Pelvic Tilt subsection in this chapter). However, true structural scoliosis is an unnatural curve of the spine in which the vertebrae themselves are rotated, resulting in the spinous processes pointing laterally instead of posteriorly. As discussed in chapter 1, muscles run from bony landmark to bony landmark; when the bony landmark moves position, the muscle is forced to work in an altered state, which is not biomechanically efficient. Because the spinal muscles run between the spinous and transverse processes at various levels (see discussion of the erector spinae and deep rotators of the spine in chapter 8), altering the arrangements of the bone leads to a variety of issues. Considering the muscles are on either side of the spine, one side may be lengthened while the other is shortened. Additional spinal considerations include the embryotic development of wedge-shaped or misshaped vertebrae and additional or missing vertebrae, which would result in dysfunctions similar to scoliosis.

Treatment of scoliosis to realign the bones is at the discretion of the treating surgeon and offers its own set of potential concerns for the patient. From a manual therapy perspective, treatment of scoliosis symptoms is a short-term plan to offer relief. For some athletes, daily self-care and treatment may be necessary for optimal performance. Information on how to treat scoliosis can be found in the appropriate treatment sections for the upper back muscles in chapter 7 and the lower back muscles in chapter 8.

LOWER LIMB-LENGTH INEQUALITY
Lower limb-length inequality (LLLI) can be either (a) functional as a result of muscle imbalance or (b) structural owing to trauma (e.g., a fracture or congenital development). The resulting dysfunction is muscle shortening on the longer leg side. This shortening can be seen anywhere on the kinetic chain, with the low back (quadratus lumborum) and lateral hip (gluteus medius) being the most likely culprits. Other compensation could be seen with the hip flexors. Although the shortened muscles side (longer leg side) often produces the symptoms, a balanced manual therapy treatment would address the lengthened muscles (found on the shorter leg side) as well. The muscles on the shorter leg side become eccentrically strained to achieve balance in the pelvis. The adjustments to an LLLI can be seen all the way up the kinetic chain with imbalance in the shoulders as well as scoliosis. A simple orthopedic insert such as a heel lift on the short side may help with the issue; however, if the person often does not wear shoes (e.g., beach volleyball players) or plays a sport in which a heel lift is not feasible (e.g., in spikes for a track athlete or cleats for a soccer player), the heel lift will not help during sport activity but could aid in performing activities of daily living. Therefore, in most cases, dysfunction will be present in the other muscles and would need to be addressed.

HEMIPELVIS ISSUES
Just as with LLLI, some individuals may have a pelvic discrepancy in which one hemipelvis (coxa bone, made up of the fused ilium, ischium, and pubis) embryologically develops smaller than the other. Termed a *small hemipelvis*, the dysfunction mimics that of a leg-length discrepancy; however, test results for a true leg-length discrepancy will be negative, because the femur and tibia would not be affected (Travell and Simons 1983). Additionally, the discrepancy will be seen when the person is seated upright correctly on the ischial tuberosity. Based on embryological development, a person with a small hemipelvis would also have facial asymmetry and a short upper arm, which should be noted in the clinical evaluation.

STRESS FRACTURES

Stress fractures result from a failure of the *osteoblasts*, which build bone, to keep up with the *osteoclasts*, which break down bone. Although stress fractures are considered more of an overuse injury, other factors such as hormonal, nutritional, or biomechanical concerns can lead to stress fractures. The fracture site, in general, is contraindicated for direct contact; however, with stress fractures, the compensatory musculature would be indicated for treatment. Because a stress fracture often is not diagnosed until healing starts, treatment may be indicated sooner than it would be for an acute fracture if the bone is stable. Additionally, if the stress fracture is treated surgically (e.g., for tibial stress fractures, sometimes hardware is placed along the bone to promote healing or treat repeated stress fractures), the bone can be assumed to be stable enough to treat. Because of the high incidence of biomechanical influences over stress fractures, myofascial release can help by adjusting how the body absorbs the stress. For example, if the tibia is involved, fascial release or trigger point release in the deep posterior compartment of the shank (as described in chapter 10) can release the crural fascia, a major attachment site for the muscles, relieving pain in the area.

BONE SPURS

Bone spurs (or *osteophytes*) are areas where the body lays down osseous tissue in a spot where there is not normally bone. Development of the extra bone can be embryological, or it could develop as a protective response to stress in the area. Typical areas of concern are the bony landmarks where the pull of the muscle creates the need for the osseus tissue. Knowing the cause of the bone spur is less important than understanding its presence, because having a bone spur is almost like having a constant irritating pebble in the tendon. From the perspective of manual therapy, it is important to avoid irritating the involved tissue while relieving pain and enhancing function. For example, bone spurs on the calcaneus can cause plantar fasciitis; plantar fasciitis is normally treated with compressive techniques, which may cause greater irritation to a client with a bone spur. A better treatment might be to release the Achilles tendon, gastrocnemius, and soleus to reduce the pull on the fascia without irritating it. Bone spurs or calcifications on the acromion process of the scapula could impinge on the supraspinatus tendon. In this case, treating the muscle belly would not cause discomfort, because it is away from the osteophyte location. Thorough understanding of anatomy can guide the clinician to decide the best course of treatment to relieve symptoms.

Examples of Common Structural Problems and Considerations of Ligaments

Ligaments are connective tissue found in the joints, connecting bone to bone. When a ligament is sprained, the fibers can be stretched (i.e., a first-degree sprain) or completely torn (i.e., a third-degree sprain). If the fibers can regenerate, they heal as scar tissue, which does not have the same composition as a ligament. When the ligament is completely torn, it may be unable to heal on its own, such as with the anterior cruciate ligament (ACL) of the knee or the ulnar collateral ligament (UCL) of the elbow; surgical repair would then be necessary. Either with healing on its own or with surgery, the musculature in the area may be asked to compensate during the healing process or because of the injury itself. Gait may change with a lower-extremity sprain; throwing mechanics may change with an upper-extremity sprain. Changes to mechanics may change how the muscles are used, leading to motor control issues or unwanted muscle and fascia changes.

ANTERIOR CRUCIATE LIGAMENT TEAR

The ACL is responsible for rotary stability in the knee. It prevents anterior translation of the tibia on the femur in a non-weight-bearing position, and it also prevents the femur from translating posteriorly in a weight-bearing position. Not repairing the ACL after a tear can lead to dysfunction in the joint and increase potential for early-onset knee osteoarthritis. Recovery and rehabilitation from ACL repair surgery can vary based on the graft type used (autograft versus allograft), the structure type (typically a tendon is used, which then changes physiologically in to a ligament), and the surgeon's postoperative instructions. That said, treatment of the area is dependent on all these variables as well.

The clinician should consider the muscles used in compensation for gait mechanics during the postinjury period and then presurgery and postsurgery until gait is retrained appropriately for that person. Treatment of the lower back, the hip, or even the shank may be part of the overall rehabilitation process. Other areas of compensation may include the contralateral hip and the upper body if the patient is using crutches, a brace, or both. Gaining full extension or flexion after surgery can be enhanced by myofascial release techniques, including the pin and stretch and spiraling of the fascia lata (chapter 9). Trigger points can be common in the quadriceps as part of recovery from surgery and in the gluteus medius because of antalgic gait (Travell and Simons 1983).

CHRONIC ANKLE INSTABILITY

Chronic ankle instability (CAI) is a multifactorial condition: It can be a structural issue related to chronic ankle sprains and maladaptive joint mechanics, or it can be a functional issue related to proprioception and strength concerns, again related to chronic ankle sprains. When the patient has a structural issue, it is considered a mechanical instability where there is excessive ankle movement due to laxity. Functional issues, however, are characterized by the sensation of giving way, related to proprioceptive or neuromuscular considerations. Treatment for CAI is dependent on the cause. Patients with mechanical CAI do well with joint mobilizations, along with myofascial treatments; those with functional CAI do well with myofascial treatments. Both conditions require rehabilitation, including emphasis on proprioception and functional exercise.

ULNAR COLLATERAL LIGAMENT TEAR

The *ulnar collateral ligament* is most often injured from repetitive valgus stress to the elbow. UCL injury is usually deemed an acute incidence. However, the injury is perpetuated by repetitive stress from upper-extremity sports, such as baseball, golf, and tennis. Typically, the ligament is repaired surgically; however, conservative non-operative treatment is also an option. Because stress on the elbow can be dissipated through the forearm muscles, myofascial treatment of the wrist flexors, which originate on the medial epicondyle, should be part of both conservative treatment and injury prevention as well as postsurgical treatment when medically approved.

Examples of Common Structural Problems and Considerations of Joints

Many joints have fibrocartilage structures, such as the menisci or labrums. These structures increase the contact area of the joint, creating a deeper socket for the bones to fit, and serve as shock absorbers. Injuries to the fibrocartilage structures can compromise joint function and lead to pain. At one time, removal of torn tissue was common; however, efforts have been made to repair these tissues to maintain joint congruency. Whether the injury is in the preoperative phase, postoperative phase, or maintenance phase, manual therapy cannot be used to treat the injured tissue; however, clinicians can provide relief to the muscles and fascia responding to the changes in the kinetic chain based on the fibrocartilage changes. The information in this section is meant to be used with chapters 6 to 10 on the individual muscles, along with the techniques outlined in chapter 3, to address the associated soft tissues compromised with the structural problems. However, clinicians are always encouraged to examine the patient and work with their goals in creating the treatment plan.

KNEE MENISCUS TEAR

There are two menisci in the knee: The *medial meniscus* is more O shaped, and the *lateral meniscus* is more U shaped. The menisci sit on the tibial plateau and provide a deeper space for the femoral condyles. Additionally, they provide shock absorption and prevent bone-on-bone contact of the tibia and femur. Meniscal tears can range from a small disruption in continuity to a large flap that flips over in the joint space. Injuries to the meniscus can result in removing a piece of the meniscus (meniscectomy) or suturing (stapling, tacking) to bring the ends together. Because parts of the menisci have poor blood supply, interventions to vascularize the area may be used to promote healing. Surgical procedures continue to evolve, so it is important for clinicians to consult with the patient's surgeon about the specific procedure if they require more information; this may be as simple as requesting the surgical notes or asking a direct question.

With any knee surgery, the patient will likely experience arthrogenic muscle inhibition, in which the quadriceps is inhibited from contracting. From a rehabilitation perspective, this is why the first exercise advised is quadriceps sets (i.e., isometric contraction of the quadriceps group). The role of the quadriceps group in controlling the patella and in eccentric control in gait is of high importance. Although many massage therapy techniques are contraindicated immediately after surgery (because of edema, open wounds, and pain), application of techniques to relieve the fascia and to address trigger points in the quadriceps becomes more important as the patient progresses through rehabilitation. Just as clinicians look to balance the vastus lateralis and vastus medialis to control movement of the patella with exercise, the use of manual therapy techniques that address the pull of the lateral structures against the weakness of the medial structures can assist in creating balance. Treatments for the distal hamstrings to improve range of motion are also indicated as part of the rehabilitation and recovery process. As with any condition in which the patient may be non-weight-bearing, treatment can focus on the hips or upper body.

SHOULDER LABRAL TEAR

The labrum of the shoulder serves to deepen the pocket of the glenoid cavity and to assist in statically controlling the head of the humerus along with the capsule. The head of the humerus is approximately three times the size of the glenoid cavity, meaning only about a third of the head sits in the cavity at a time. Correct positioning of the humeral head is similar to lining up a golf ball on a tee. When the labrum is torn, some of the static stability is lost, and the head of the humerus can be knocked off its proverbial tee. Additionally, the long head of the biceps brachii has an attachment into the labrum, leading to muscle insufficiency when the labrum is torn away from the bone in the area of the biceps brachii tendon attachment.

Although the labrum, along with the capsule, provides static constraint, the rotator cuff muscles provide dynamic constraint as they function to control the humeral head in the glenoid cavity. Although rotator cuff tendon issues (addressed in chapter 6) can lead to dysfunction, labral tears can lead to rotator cuff tendinopathies as a compensatory response (making rotator cuff injuries a secondary injury). Additional functional issues of scapula misalignment (caused by functional concerns) can also put stress on the labrum. With the shoulder, the scenario becomes one of which-came-first.

Treatment when the labrum is torn (before repair) should first focus on relieving the areas of patient concern as well as the muscles that will be influenced by the requirements of the sport. There is no set treatment in this scenario because the starting place is arbitrary. Depending on the sport and time of year, the patient may require manual therapy for a prolonged period before surgery occurs, especially if they are still able to participate. After surgery, it is important to follow the postsurgical guidelines for range of motion and immobilization. Once the patient is out of the sling, however, manual therapy can be used to assist with releasing the fascia of the internal rotators shortened by the position of immobilization. Manual therapy will continue to be an important part of the rehabilitation and treatment process to assist the patient in gaining range of motion and strength as well as regaining sport-specific skills.

HIP LABRAL TEAR

The labrum of the hip serves the same purpose as the labrum of the shoulder: to increase surface area and provide some shock absorption. The acetabulum in the hip is a much deeper socket, and the head of the femur is much more stable than the head of the humerus. Dislocation and subluxation are less common in the hip, and labral tears are less of a cause of instability. However, tears in the labrum cause pain and impingement. Additional considerations are based on the person's structure; for example, the acetabulum may be shallow or even too deep to allow for correct movement of the head. Over time, some people may develop bony growths (bone spurs), which may impinge on movement.

The entire scope of issues at the hip is more than can be comprehensively understood in this short paragraph, and diagnosis of such would require imaging. Regardless of the cause of the dysfunction, any situation involving hip joint pain and compromised movement will have a similar effect on the muscles. Much of the hip pain will be felt anteriorly, right in the crease in the hip. A few structures may cause pain in that area, which is most likely referred pain from the deeper hip joint. From a fascial perspective, the fascia lata gathers superiorly right in that space, creating the inguinal ligament (see chapter 1). Pain and dysfunction in the hip can alter the pull of the fascia lata (remember the concept of tensegrity in chapter 1), leading to this pull and pinch in the inguinal crease. A second cause of pain in that area, either related to injury or postoperatively, is the indirect head of the rectus femoris, which originates at the acetabulum and a bit of the capsule of the hip (see chapter 9 for the muscle origin). Especially with surgery when the capsule is compromised to reach the deeper structures, the patient may experience discomfort in the rectus femoris, resulting in some myofascial pain and trigger points. Superficially, two other muscles cross in that area of the hip: the sartorius and the tensor fasciae latae. More deeply, the pectineus and the adductor longus create the femoral triangle. Specific manual therapy techniques for the hip flexors and adductors are warranted for this condition, regardless of whether it is from the labrum or bony abnormalities.

Examples of Common Structural Problems and Considerations of the Spine

Some additional considerations for the spine may compromise positioning of the vertebrae, which will, in turn, lead to alterations in the muscles and fascia and their responses to stress. Any muscle that attaches to the vertebrae can be compromised based on the positioning of the vertebra of its origin or insertion. Any condition that alters or compromises the spaces between the vertebrae can also be a structural change. Some of these deviations may be permanent structural changes, or they could be related to a pathology that resolves itself over time.

SPINAL CURVATURES

The spine has four distinct curves: two anterior or lordotic curves and two posterior or kyphotic curves. The two kyphotic curves, found in the thoracic and sacral regions, are primary curves, developing embryologically. The two lordotic curves, found in the cervical and lumbar regions, develop secondary to upright gait. Imagine a baby engaged in tummy time: This position forces the baby to lift his head, strengthening his posterior musculature and assisting in creating the cervical lordotic curve. As the baby develops strength in his core, he will begin to crawl and eventually attempt upright gait. The movement of the upper body into the erect posture helps create the second lordotic curve in the lumbar region. The purpose of these curves is to efficiently distribute forces during movements. Although humans create these good curves early in life, their habits later in life can lead to overexaggeration of the anterior curve (a lordosis) or overexaggeration of the posterior curve (a kyphosis). Additionally, a loss of either of these curves can lead to dysfunction. Although manual therapy can be used to relieve pain and muscle tightness associated with these conditions, strengthening the muscles, improving flexibility and range of motion, and adjusting poor postural or ergonomic habits can help to alleviate pain and potentially restore normal spinal curves.

DISC PATHOLOGY

In the space between each of the vertebra from C2 to S1 is an intervertebral disc. These discs are made of fibrocartilage, with a stronger outer annulus fibrosus and a gelatinous center, termed the *nucleus pulposus*. These discs are part of the shock absorption and force distribution system, along with the curves in the spine. As the cervical region progresses to the lumbar region, the discs become larger and thicker, because they are responsible for absorbing greater amounts of force. Loss of fluid from the discs can decrease the space between vertebrae. Pressure on the discs can lead to weakening of the annulus fibrosus. If the nucleus pulposus is compressed, it may begin to push into the annulus fibrosus and potentially leak out or herniate into the annulus fibrosus. Additionally, the disc can push out into space and compress the spinal nerves at the individual segment, leading to numbness and tingling or a decrease in motor function.

Disc pathology has many potential issues and concerns, making treatment more complex than captured in the scope of this text. No amount of manual therapy can fix a disc pathology. As with other conditions, manual therapy can be used to relieve muscle tension and some of the secondary symptoms. However, patients should consult a physician before treatment to ensure manual therapy is not contraindicated for their condition. Caution should be taken if sensation is compromised, because the patient may not be able to adequately provide feedback on the pressure. Movement with treatment should be avoided if it has the potential to exacerbate symptoms, particularly in the cervical region.

Functional Issues

Functional considerations are related to the muscles or fascia (figure 4.2). Some functional considerations can be adjusted for optimal levels; others are related to sport and may need to be worked within limits but not eliminated. It is important for clinicians to have a good understanding of anatomy to know which muscles may be functionally stressed by a sport. It is not as important for clinicians to be experts in a sport before they work with an athlete. Clinicians should ask athletes to show them what they are experiencing, and they should use their knowledge of anatomy and techniques to problem-solve.

Manual therapy is one way to assist with functional deficiencies. Other options include stretching and strengthening. As outlined with the postural and phasic

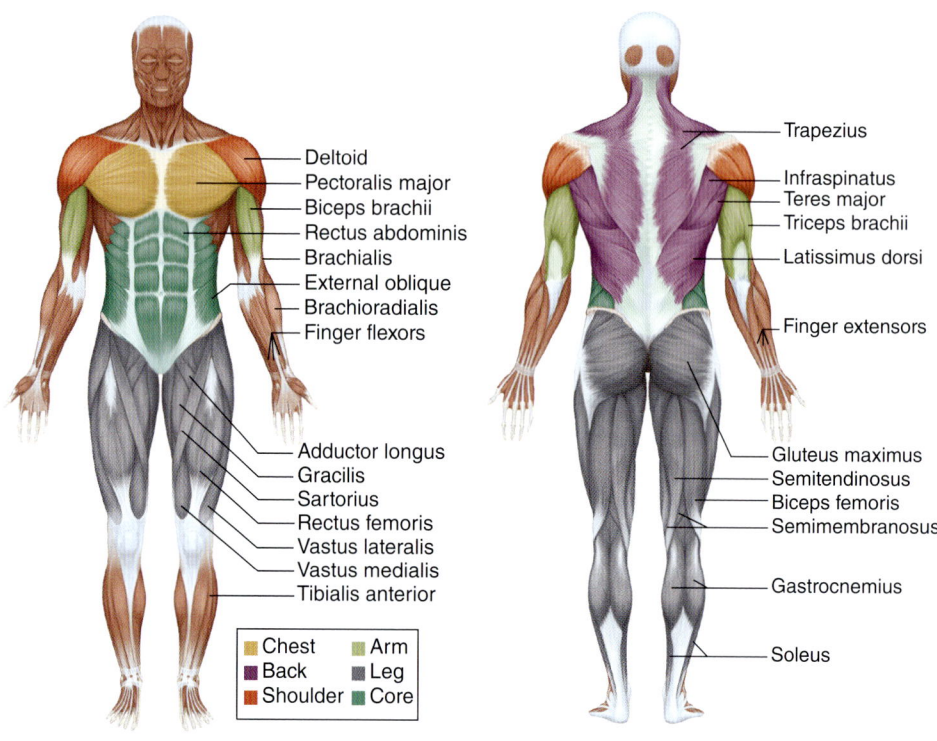

Figure 4.2 Conditions related to the muscles or fascia are functional and can be positively influenced by manual therapy; however, in sports, some functional adjustments will remain while the person continues to be involved in their sport.

muscles in chapter 1, clinicians should provide the appropriate care depending on the muscle type and the issues presented. More information on home self-care is provided in chapter 11, but specific strengthening treatments are not covered in this book.

Examples of Common Functional Problems and Considerations of the Shoulder

Because the shoulder is highly mobile and reliant on the muscles to have optimal structural function, there are many overlaps between functional and structural considerations of the shoulder. In fact, it may be difficult to differentiate between functional and structural problems, and the structural issues might be investigated only if the functional approach does not work. Many of the limitations in the shoulder come directly from the positioning of the scapula, which will determine the position of the glenoid cavity that will, in turn, determine the position of the humerus. Misalignment at these levels will alter the mechanics of activities involving the upper extremity. In this case, the goal of manual therapy is to balance the postural and phasic muscles, whereas the goal of rehabilitation is to provide appropriate strength balance to maintain adequate scapular positioning. More details will be presented in chapter 6.

ROTATOR CUFF

The *rotator cuff* is made up of four muscles: the supraspinatus, infraspinatus, teres minor, and subscapularis. Their tendons not only keep the head of the humerus in the glenoid cavity, but they also keep it moving correctly in the cavity for optimal movement. Although the rotator cuff is subject to various pathologies ranging from impingement to tendinopathy to strains, the manual therapy treatment remains similar. The rotator cuff muscles will need to be treated for any trigger points or fascial restrictions. The scapular stabilizers must be balanced with the scapular retractors and protractors (discussed next). Along with balance from a manual therapy perspective, there needs to be a balance with strength and endurance. Without proper rehabilitation, the manual therapy treatment will not be enough to show improvement.

PROTRACTED SHOULDER

A *protracted shoulder*, or rounded shoulder, is a postural position in which the scapula is abducted (away from the spine), resulting in misalignment of the shoulder joint as the glenoid cavity moves more anteriorly. This movement results in a more anterior and potentially internally rotated humerus. The muscles of the anterior aspect of the shoulder, specifically the protractors (pectoralis minor and serratus anterior), are postural and respond to stress by shortening. For most people, daily habits and activities result in positioning the arms in horizontal adduction and flexion, which forces the scapula to be abducted. Based on Davis' law (discussed in chapter 1), the more time people spend with the scapulae protracted, the more likely the scapular retractors, rhomboids, and middle trapezius will elongate, lay down more connective tissue, and weaken. As a result, the position of the scapula can change and thus cause dysfunction over time, as outlined earlier with rotator cuff pathologies.

It is not unusual for a client to present with upper back pain and feel like those muscles need to be stretched. These muscles are, in fact, not tight but taut like a drum, and techniques used to balance the scapula alignment are indicated. The muscle fibers of the scapular retractors are eccentrically loaded and strained, resulting in the upper back pain. Releasing these muscles is better served by stretching the anterior chest (pectoralis major and pectoralis minor), thereby relieving and relaxing the posterior musculature. Continued anterior stretching combined with strengthening the posterior muscles, adjusting ergonomics, taking breaks, and receiving manual therapy treatment are all good ways to relieve these muscles.

BICEPS BRACHII TENDINOPATHY

Typically, *biceps brachii tendinopathy* affects one or both origins of the muscle, where it acts on the shoulder joint. As indicated earlier and in chapter 6, the long head of the biceps brachii has an attachment at the supraglenoid tubercle of the scapula and into the labrum of the shoulder and comes through the bicipital groove. The attachment places the tendon of the long head of the biceps brachii at risk of inflammation and increases potential for one of the various diagnoses of tendinopathy, including snapping of the tendon in the bicipital groove. The short head attaches to the coracoid process, a biomechanically stressed area of the shoulder, subjecting the tendon of the short head of the biceps brachii to inflammation and tendinopathy related to the protracted shoulder. Because of these crossovers, biceps brachii tendinopathy may be diagnosed first, but it is paramount to determine whether there is a primary cause. Treating only the symptoms of biceps brachii tendinopathy will not solve the underlying problem. However, much of the treatment may cross over to the treatments of the primary cause.

Examples of Common Functional Problems and Considerations of the Neck and Upper Back

The common functional problems of the neck and upper back build on the common problems of the shoulder. As mentioned earlier, the primary complaint of upper back pain often is related to a protracted scapula and a rounded shoulder posture. There is also a similar relationship with the rounded shoulder posture and forward head posture. Therefore, although this text chooses to break things down from this perspective, it is not wrong to combine functional conditions of the neck and upper back with the shoulder, creating an upper-body protocol.

FORWARD HEAD POSTURE

Forward head posture involves shortening of the cervical extensors and lengthening of the cervical flexors. In this case, the head moves away from sitting directly on the cervical vertebrae, which can result in a straightening of the normal lordotic curve in the cervical spine. From the side, the ear canal (external auditory meatus) should line up with the acromioclavicular joint of the shoulder. With forward head posture, inspection from the lateral view will reveal the head forward of that line. As a secondary compensation to the forward head, the atlantooccipital joint (the occiput and C1) will be hyperextended. Because the body is inclined to look at the horizon, dubbed the *righting reflex*, the suboccipital muscles that run between the occiput, C1, and C2 can shorten or become compressed and respond with trigger points in response to this hyperextension.

SCAPULAR MISPOSITIONING

Scapular mispositioning can include any variety of situations in which the scapula deviates from its normal perspective. Although this could be included with protracted scapulae (as described earlier), where from the posterior perspective the scapulae are viewed as being abducted and positioned away from their normal alignment with the spine, that is not the only potential misalignment. Scapular protraction often is a bilateral phenomenon, as it would be with a rounded shoulder posture; however, the scapulae are not required to move equally bilaterally. Consider the example of an athlete in a throwing sport: Her dominant shoulder may move differently than the nondominant side. In this case, her dominant side could be strong and have appropriate muscle movement, whereas her nondominant side may be weaker and show a lack of anterior or posterior balance. There may be no dysfunction in the side used for her sport, and there may not even be any complaints from the nondominant side, but the postural asymmetry may be noted. Also, in a condition such as scapular dyskinesis, fatigue may cause the dysfunction, and scapular asymmetry may only appear when the person is fatigued.

UPPER CROSS SYNDROME

Upper cross syndrome is a combination of forward head posture, rounded shoulders, and protracted scapula (figure 4.3). With this combination of postural and phasic muscles, the lengthened and shortened structures cross. The chest muscles, including the pectoralis major and the pectoralis minor, are short and tight, whereas the lower trapezius and the serratus anterior are weakened and lengthened. The anterior neck (the cervical spine flexors) becomes weakened and lengthened, whereas the posterior neck (the upper portion of the trapezius and the levator scapulae) is shortened. These distortions are common based on someone's everyday habits, which may or may not be exacerbated by sport-specific activities. In fact, for clinicians working with student athletes who are balancing classroom work with sport and for those working with recreational athletes with a desk job, habits that develop from working on a computer or other device may be as much of a contributing factor as sport. Addressing these concerns would involve discussing ways to improve ergonomics and create balancing habits.

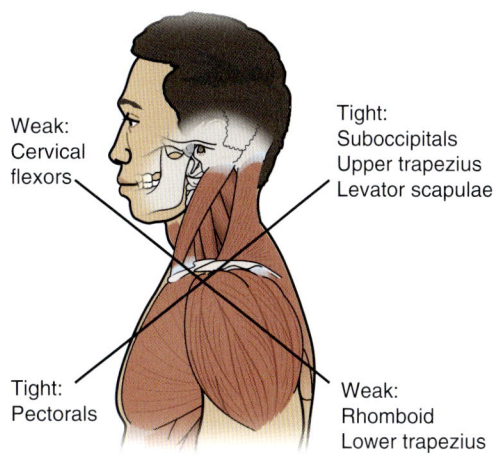

Figure 4.3 Upper cross syndrome is characterized by shortened and tight anterior chest and posterior head muscles and lengthened and weak anterior neck and posterior thoracic muscles.

Examples of Common Functional Problems and Considerations of the Low Back

Problems with the low back typically start with changes to the lumbar musculature. Many concerns with the back tend to be related to the musculature. Like the shoulder, muscle dysfunction can cause structural changes (e.g., changes to the normal lordotic and kyphotic curves) or can result from structural changes (e.g., scoliosis). Between the lower ribs and the iliac crest, there is only soft tissue, muscle, and fascia; therefore, a lack of strength, flexibility, or symmetry can lead to dysfunction and pain. Therefore, manual therapy treatments, along with stretching and improved range of motion, can be integral in relieving low back pain that stems from the myofascial system.

LOW BACK PAIN

Low back pain is a descriptive term without any diagnostic criteria and potentially without a clear mechanism of injury or known cause. General low back pain often stems from a musculature imbalance. As indicated in the Structural Issues section in this chapter and in the discussion of the low back musculature in chapter 8, altered positions of the vertebra based on structural changes can lead to pain. Spasm or dysfunction in the muscle may also alter the position of the vertebrae. In that case, muscular dysfunction leads to low back pain. Additional functional considerations include low back spasms, mismatch in strength from one side to the other, or deficiencies in range of motion.

LATERAL PELVIC TILT

Lateral pelvic tilt can be seen in the frontal plane and is characterized by the iliac crest on one side being higher than the iliac crest on the other side (figure 4.4). It does not matter which side is higher because even if the higher side is more painful, the lower side may be the side of dysfunction. In this case, a lateral cross is seen where the quadratus lumborum is shortened on the high side and lengthened (or normal) on the low side. The ipsilateral gluteus medius is lengthened on the high side with the shortened quadratus lumborum, and the contralateral gluteus medius is shortened on the lower side with the lengthened (or normal) quadratus lumborum. In this case, the balance is side to side as opposed to anterior to posterior. Additionally, this compensation may be seen with one raised shoulder, which will also cause a lean to the short side. The raised shoulder often comes from carrying a bag on one side, and the contralateral quadratus lumborum will be shortened with lateral flexion of the spine occurring to the contralateral side.

Examples of Common Functional Problems and Considerations of the Hip

Considerations of the hip for structural issues center around the acetabulofemoral joint—the true hip joint. However, when functional issues are

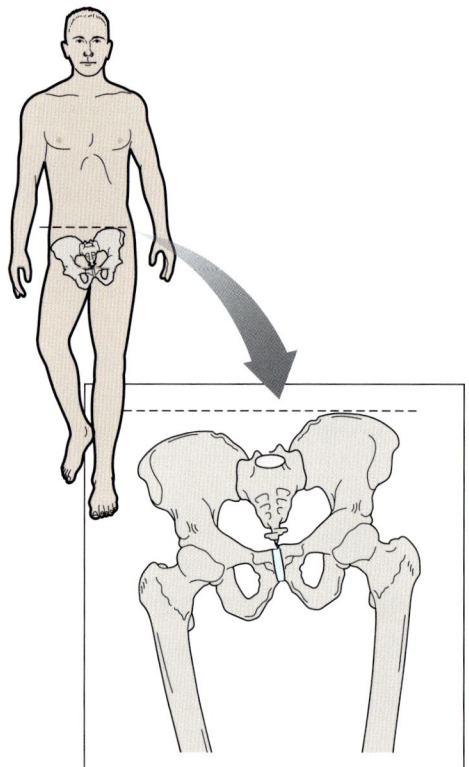

Figure 4.4 Lateral pelvic tilt is characterized by one side being short, with the iliac crest being higher on one side, and the other side being lengthened, with the iliac crest being lower or even in its normal orientation.

identified, the sacroiliac joint and the pubic symphysis must also be considered. The muscles that produce movement at the hip originate on the ilium, ischium, and pubic bones; therefore, these regions will be addressed during manual therapy treatment. Additionally, the position of the pelvis can be pulled in the direction of the shortened muscles, as described in the following subsection on anterior pelvic tilt (with the hip flexors pulling the pelvis anteriorly) or in the previous section on lateral pelvic tilt (which can be caused by the quadratus lumborum, gluteus medius, or gluteus minimus).

ANTERIOR PELVIC TILT

Anterior pelvic tilt is characterized by the pelvis sitting in a position such that the anterior superior iliac spine drops lower than the posterior superior iliac spine, two bony landmarks that are level in a balanced pelvis. In this condition, the pelvis is rotated such that the ischial tuberosity points more posteriorly than inferiorly. From a muscle perspective, anterior pelvic tilt is characterized by tight hip flexors, in which the insertion on the femur is stable and the origin on the pelvis or low back (in the case of the psoas major) is closer to the origin than in a normal postural position. This condition can be caused by a musculature imbalance, such as tight and shortened hip flexors, but it can also come from abdominal distention, such as with pregnancy or excessive adipose tissue in that area. Habits such as wearing high-heeled shoes or spending substantial time in a seated position can lead to short and tight hip flexors. An anterior pelvic tilt can be bilateral, where both sides are forward, or it can be unilateral, where one side appears more rotated.

LOWER CROSS SYNDROME

Lower cross syndrome, like upper cross syndrome, is an imbalance of muscles from anterior to posterior, superior to inferior (figure 4.5). In the case of lower cross syndrome, the tight musculature is found in the hip flexors and the lower erectors, resulting in an anterior pelvic tilt and an excessive lordotic curve (*lordosis*) in the lumbar spine. The lengthened muscles are the upper portion of the hamstrings (the attachment to the ischial tuberosity that functions as a hip extender) and the abdominal muscles. Unlike an anterior pelvic tilt, the contribution comes from all areas of the cross and requires muscle rebalancing. However, if an anterior pelvic tilt remains untreated, it is possible the rest of the muscles will follow into lower cross syndrome.

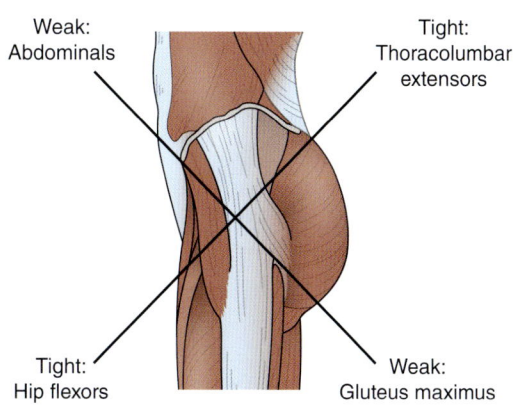

Figure 4.5 Lower cross syndrome is characterized by tight and shortened hip flexors and low back muscles accompanied by weak and lengthened abdominal muscles and hip extenders.

PIRIFORMIS SYNDROME

Piriformis syndrome and sciatica are often misrepresented as the same condition. *Sciatica* directly affects the sciatic nerve, which is outside the scope of this book. In *piriformis syndrome*, the piriformis responds to stress as a postural muscle by shortening and widening. The sciatic nerve runs deep to the piriformis, and a short and wide piriformis can put pressure on the sciatic nerve, eliciting neurological symptoms of numbness and tingling as well as weakness. Additionally, poor seated posture that involves sitting on the gluteal region (posterior pelvic tilt), instead of sitting up straight on the ischial tuberosity, can lead to compression of both the piriformis and sciatic nerve. In addition, keeping something in a back pocket, such as a wallet or phone, can lead to unilateral compression of the piriformis and sciatic nerve. Because the piriformis is a postural muscle, it needs to be lengthened (stretched). However, because the sciatic nerve is compressed in piriformis syndrome and the most common manual therapy technique used involves compression of the piriformis muscle, it is important to consider a different technique if the patient has neurological symptoms.

Examples of Common Functional Problems and Considerations of the Knee

Many conditions affecting the knee joint (the condyles of the femur resting on the tibial plateau) are more structural, from meniscal tears to ligament reconstruction to total knee replacement. Functional concerns can center more around the patellofemoral joint and how the patella glides in the femoral groove, because the patella is controlled by the quadriceps tendon. Imbalance between the medial and lateral myofascial structures, with typically the lateral side providing more of the pull, can cause much of the knee pain. For these problems, balancing the medial and lateral structures is a large part of decreasing pain.

PATELLAR TRACKING CONCERNS (PATELLOFEMORAL PAIN SYNDROME)

Patellofemoral pain syndrome is a collection of nonspecific symptoms related to the tracking of the patella in the groove between the femoral condyles. Because of the shape of the posterior aspect of the patella, the facets on the posterior patella (specifically, the odd facet) when the patella is not tracking correctly produce a bone-on-bone condition that can be painful and can lead to osteochondral changes if left untreated. The quadriceps, specifically the vastus lateralis and the vastus medialis, are responsible for guiding patellar tracking. Lack of balance between the vastus lateralis, which is much larger and therefore stronger, and the vastus medialis, which is typically weaker, leads to the patella being pulled more laterally. Releasing the tight lateral structures, including the iliotibial (IT) band, along with strengthening the vastus medialis helps keep the patella in the correct line of pull, thereby decreasing forces on the posterior side of the patella.

ILIOTIBIAL BAND SYNDROME

The IT band is not a separate structure from the fascia lata; rather, it is an overlap or thickening of the fascia on the lateral aspect of the thigh. The fascia lata is controlled by the dynamic fibers of the tensor fasciae latae (the muscle), which are encased in the fascia lata. *Iliotibial band syndrome* has many potential causes, but they all center around a combination of flexion at the hip and knee in repetitive movement, such as seen with distance runners and cyclists. Tightness can originate at either the hip or knee, making the most effective treatment one that occurs at both the hip and knee, regardless of where the pain originates. Additional considerations that can lead to IT band syndrome may be structural or functional. These considerations include leg-length discrepancies, which force the hip into a lateral pelvic tilt (see earlier section on lateral pelvic tilt), as well as hyperpronation of the foot (see the Hyperpronation subsection), training on uneven surfaces, and running curves (e.g., on a track).

PES ANSERINE TENDINOSIS

The *pes anserine,* (which translates to goose's foot) is a common attachment site for the tendons of three muscles: the sartorius, gracilis, and semitendinosus. Because these muscles pull in three different directions with their actions, the area can become irritated and inflamed, leading to any one of the tendinous pathologies. Direct massage over the area may lead to more inflammation. However, treatment of the muscle may allow for relief in the area.

Examples of Common Functional Problems and Considerations of the Low Leg and Foot

The instructor of my first clinical anatomy course would often say, "When the foot hits the ground, everything changes." Although much of anatomy including the actions of muscles is described from an open-chain position in which the limb is free to move and not fixed to a surface, the lower extremity functions in a closed-chain position in which the foot is fixed against a surface, typically the ground. For this reason, structural and functional considerations of the foot will influence the myofascial system. Thus, there is always a balance between addressing the myofascial chain and the structural components, while not changing gait too much to create "normal" when these adjustments may lead to ineffective movements.

MEDIAL TIBIAL STRESS SYNDROME

Medial tibial stress syndrome (MTSS) involves pain along the medial border of the tibia. This condition usually results from running, but it can also be caused by jumping or exacerbated by increasing activity too quickly. MTSS is a catchall term for pain in the low leg, and it is sometimes incorrectly referred to as *shin splints*. There are different theories on the exact mechanism and cause of MTSS; however, they all lead back to myofascial pain from the deep posterior compartment of the muscles, typically the tibialis posterior, and the associated crural fascia. Manual therapy can be applied to this area to relieve trigger points and release the fascia, thereby decreasing pain.

ACHILLES TENDINOSIS

The Achilles tendon is the distal attachment of the gastrocnemius and soleus into the calcaneus. Because the gastrocnemius and soleus are postural muscles, they are short and tight, resulting in plantar flexion and potentially restricting dorsiflexion. When the Achilles tendon is irritated (*Achilles tendinosis*), treatment involves stretching and lengthening the plantar flexors. Habits such as wearing shoes with a heel or running on the toes can shorten the Achilles tendon and lead to plantar flexion as the normal resting position. Additionally, the dorsiflexors are not as large or as strong as the plantar flexors, leading to a positioning mismatch when someone is in a non-weight-bearing position. Manual therapy application to the gastrocnemius and soleus, along with stretching and rehabilitation, can assist in treating this condition.

PLANTAR FASCIITIS

Plantar fasciitis involves inflammation of the fascia on the plantar surface of the foot. This condition is characterized by pain when first stepping down in the morning and pain along the heel. The plantar fascia attaches to the calcaneal tubercle, the same attachment site as the Achilles tendon, and functions as both a spring to propel the body forward and as a shock absorber for the weight of the body during gait. Plantar fasciitis can be caused by several factors, including incorrect footwear, structural foot problems, overuse, and other issues. Identifying the cause can help with manual therapy treatment. In the absence of finding the cause, symptoms can be treated with manual therapy and self-care.

HYPERPRONATION

Hyperpronation occurs when the medial longitudinal arch of the foot collapses in a weight-bearing position. It is important to note that with gait, the transition from pronation to supination is a normal part of foot movement. Therefore, pronation or being a pronator itself is not a cause for concern. Excessive pronation (hyperpronation) is an issue, because collapsing of the arch leads to secondary distortion at the knee, hip, low back, shoulders, and so on. It is fitting to end with this as a functional concern, because all the conditions listed earlier in this section can be caused by what is occurring at the plantar surface of the foot.

Biomechanically Stressed Areas and Bony Landmarks

Muscles cross the joints where they act and span from bony landmark to bony landmark. When the muscle is aligned appropriately from landmark to landmark, it can achieve the optimal line of pull for efficient contraction. In addition, the landmarks provide a road map for treating the muscles. From an anatomy perspective, having the ability to palpate for a landmark gives clinicians the confidence that they are treating the correct muscle. Throughout chapters 6 to 10, the location of the muscle attachments will be emphasized.

The bony landmarks are not apparent on the bones from birth. The force of the muscle on the bone initiates a series of physiological changes in the bone where the bone adapts to the stress put on it, forming the landmarks (*Wolf's law*). The greater the stress, the larger the area of bone. This change in bone can be seen in conditions such as Osgood-Schlatter disease, in which the tibial tuberosity becomes more prominent. However, it can also be seen as a normal adaptation when someone increases the stress in their normal routine, such as with the progression of weight training or endurance training.

Many of the bony landmarks serve as attachments for multiple muscles. In some cases, such as with the forearm flexors on the medial epicondyle of the humerus, the attachments merge to form a common tendon (one tendon for multiple separate muscles). In other cases, the muscles pull in a variety of directions, such as the coracoid process of the scapula where the pectoralis minor, short head of the biceps brachii, and coracobrachialis converge. When the muscle pull is in opposing directions, a biomechanically stressed area is created; this can result in some tenderness to touch in that area (e.g., I always know I am on the coracoid process and palpating with enough pressure when I get the telltale wince, especially from anatomy students). In an area such as the pes anserine, the pull can lead to tendinosis or to bursitis if a bursa is present.

Recognition of these biomechanically stressed areas and the muscles that attach can assist in creating a treatment plan to balance the pull of the muscles. For example, the pectoralis minor is a common cause of complaint in a rounded shoulder posture or upper cross syndrome, whereas the coracobrachialis is typically not considered. However, to create a balanced treatment, the clinician should examine the coracobrachialis for potential issues in the muscle.

WHY DOES THE CLINICIAN CARE?

There are reasons for clinicians to look at both structural and functional concerns when developing a manual therapy treatment plan. Understanding the goal of a structural problem helps the clinician to relieve myofascial pain resulting from an issue that cannot necessarily be fixed. It can be frustrating for both the clinician and the patient to not see improvement: Both should keep in mind that the goal of manual therapy treatment of structural problems is relief (albeit temporary) and not a fix. There may be a time and place for the structural problem to resolve, but most likely, the issue needs to be managed. Although functional problems seem easier to manage, they, too, can have their frustrations. Lack of progress with what appears to be functional in nature could be indicative of an underlying structural issue. In the case of an athlete, the functional issue may not resolve itself until the person finishes their competitive career. In the case of occupational athletes whose dysfunction originates from their job, it also is not as simple as stopping the offending action, because it is a source of their livelihood. The situation of not stopping an activity is especially true for tactical athletes in a military, law enforcement, or fire occupation. Many cannot stop their activities and, more importantly, may not want to change their career.

Common Compensations in Sport

Each sport or activity has common stressors. One key to working with athletes is to understand the actions necessary to be successful in sport and how the muscles may be stressed. It is outside the scope of this text to give examples of the specific stressors for each sport. However, this book provides some direction as to what clinicians might see to help them align clinical decision-making with sport-specific movements.

The goal in athlete care is to work within the biomechanically stressed areas, because clinicians will not be able to eliminate the stress produced by the sport. This goal is different from working with a client with an active injury or a patient with poor postural habits that can be corrected (e.g., fixing seated posture at a desk or adjusting seat positioning in a car). Clinicians cannot tell a baseball pitcher not to throw or a tennis player to balance their dominant and nondominant sides. The differences were created in response to sport, and fixing something that is not broken may lead to injury down the line.

Considerations also must be made for performing artists and tactical athletes, who may not have traditional sport seasons. Performing artists may have daily practices and daily performances, with little time off to recover, relying on techniques that can keep them active daily. Tactical or occupational athletes, including military members, police officers, and firefighters, require a high level of physical performance for their job and may have additional stressors, such as long shifts and lack of sleep, that contribute to their performance concerns. Clothing or equipment worn for an occupation, such as costumes for performing artists or duty belts for police officers, can create muscular imbalances because individuals must adapt to the added weight, which may not be equally distributed. These populations rely on their physical performance for both their occupation and their livelihood, meaning they may be subject to workers' compensation laws and agreements if they suffer an injury at work. In addition, the culture of these groups may tend toward continuing to work while hurt, which the clinician must consider as part of the manual therapy treatment. Loss of livelihood and identity is common in these groups as much as with the athlete population.

Upper-Extremity Stressors

Examination of upper-extremity sport stressors typically starts with the throwing athlete. The shoulder joint coordination (outlined in chapter 6) and the energy transfer from the lower extremity through the core into the upper extremity required to throw consistently can be influenced by any dysfunction in the myofascial system. This section focuses on the upper extremity, but clinicians may refer to the Lower-Extremity Stressors section if dysfunction in the kinetic chain seems to occur elsewhere. Other overhead athletes, such as swimmers, tennis players, and even those who do overhead weightlifting, are discussed separately, although the mechanics used in throwing may apply. Finally, considerations for athletes who rely on grip strength, such as tennis players, softball pitchers, and pickleball players, are described. Again, this chapter overlaps with chapters 4 and 6 in discussing the upper extremity, which is intentional in the organization of this book.

Throwing Athletes

To achieve both force and accuracy when throwing, the body must go through a precise and coordinated sequence of movements from the ground up. The lower half of the body and the core initiate the movement, not the shoulder or arm. Relying on or using too much of the arm not only results in a poor throw, but over time it also leads to myofascial dysfunction and injury. Once the ball is released, slowing of the arm and adequate follow-through are essential to reduce stress on the shoulder. If the muscles are unable to slow the arm down, the stresses will be felt into the joint structure.

Phases of throwing follow this order: wind-up, stride, cocking, acceleration, deceleration, and follow-through (figure 5.1). Although the actual mechanics of throwing are outside the scope of this text, it is important for clinicians to know the terms related to these phases when working with athletes and coaches. Ask the patient when they experience pain coordinated with the various phases; or, if more appropriate, request that the patient show where in the movement they are experiencing pain. Combine this information with having them point to the corresponding location of the pain on their body. Answers to such questions can help the clinician develop the treatment plan by combining the mechanics with a working knowledge of anatomy. Effective throwing is a coordination of the aforementioned movements, firing of the muscles, and range of motion. Structural issues (e.g., labral tears) and functional issues (e.g., protracted scapula) will not

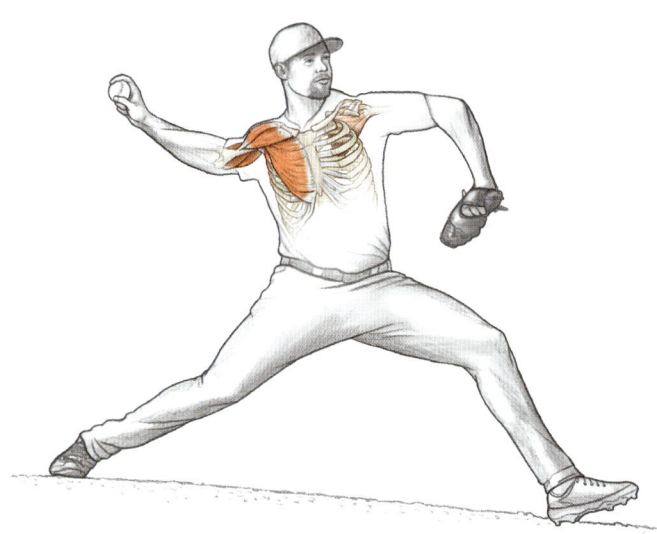

Figure 5.1 The cocking phase of throwing with potential energy harnessed in the muscles from the shoulder through the core and the legs.

allow for correct and coordinated movement, as discussed in chapter 4. Select myofascial issues related to throwing mechanics are outlined here.

When the clinician is observing the patient in the cocking phase, the range of motion (specifically, transverse plane movements of rotation and horizontal adduction) should also be examined. A maximum of 150 to 180 degrees of external rotation is needed during this phase (Mayes et al. 2022). Excess external rotation can lead to diminished strength, because the muscles will not be aligned correctly to execute the contraction cycle effectively (see discussion of the sliding filament theory in chapter 1). Less external rotation will not allow for enough force generation. When creating a treatment plan, clinicians should remember this range to provide the appropriate stretching protocol; stretching a client with an excess of 180 degrees of external rotation would not be warranted.

In addition to rotation, approximately 20 degrees of horizontal adduction is needed to bring the shoulder into the correct position while allowing for the pectoralis major and the anterior deltoid to optimally produce enough angular velocity for the throw (Mayes et al. 2022). Lack of flexibility in the anterior shoulder can prevent enough range of motion to reach optimal efficiency. The deceleration phase requires eccentric control of the posterior muscle chain and use of the anterior arm muscles (biceps brachii and brachialis) to control the anterior arm (Mayes et al. 2022). Because of the emphasis on the posterior rotator cuff and the posterior axioscapular muscles in the deceleration process, proper positioning of the scapula is necessary. To prevent scapular dyskinesis, these muscles also must be able to withstand the fatigue of multiple throws, especially in later stages of a game. With all this information, clinicians should keep in mind the laws of exercise physiology, in which range of motion can be negatively affected by trigger points or lack of balance in the agonist–antagonist relationship.

Overhead Sports

Any activity involving consistent overhead use of the arm can result in excess stress on the shoulder if the scapulohumeral rhythm is not balanced (see chapter 6 for more about scapulohumeral rhythm). This subsection is dedicated to any overhead motion in sport that is not throwing, such as hitting a volleyball, swimming, serving in tennis, reaching up to catch a pass in football, or shooting a basketball. As soon as the arm is raised, the position of the scapula must be altered to allow for more space between the acromion and the head of the humerus. The shoulder joints allow for increased mobility, but stability is sacrificed in return. Manual therapies, along with appropriate strengthening, can be used to help maintain balance between the postural and phasic muscles.

As seen with the throwing athlete, there is a balance between strength and range of motion. Too much range of motion will diminish the ability to harness potential energy into strength. Too little range of motion can cause other areas of the kinetic chain to pick up the slack and become stressed, leading to fatigue or injury. For example, a lack of external rotation in the shoulder may increase rotation of the spine, causing the back muscles to fatigue sooner. Therefore, it is always important for the clinician to examine the entire kinetic chain in treatment.

Grip-Related Stressors

Some sports have grip-related stressors. For example, in racket sports (e.g., tennis and pickleball), the forearm muscles are engaged from multiple perspectives. As discussed in chapter 6, the forearm muscles include extrinsic muscles involved in finger flexion (on the anterior aspect of the forearm) and finger extension (on the posterior aspect of the forearm). These muscles also double as wrist flexors and extensors, respectively (figure 5.2). When the muscles are asked to engage in multiple actions (e.g., flexion of the fingers and flexion of the wrist), the muscles are not efficient in both actions at the same time: They cannot generate enough force to produce both actions, which is termed *active insufficiency*. Additionally, when the wrist is extended, the extrinsic finger flexors become

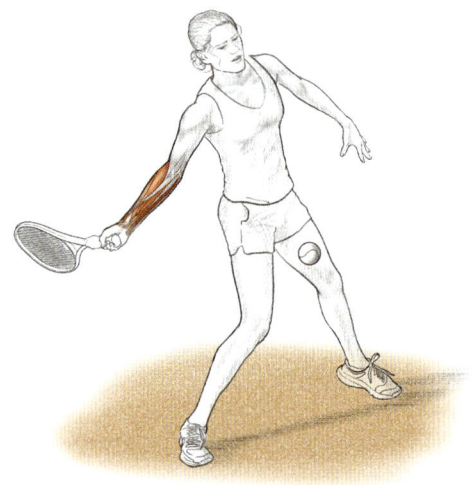

Figure 5.2 In racket sports, the muscles of the forearm are used for gripping as well as flexion and extension of the wrist during forehand and backhand shots, respectively.

lengthened. When the person flexes the fingers around the handle of a racket (or paddle or bat), the forearm flexors become a victim of passive insufficiency. Either can lead to myofascial pain or trigger points in the forearm muscles.

Additional concerns for forearm pain can include any activity that involves grip strength, engaging the fingers as well as flexion or extension of the forearm. Sport activities can include baseball or softball, in which players use grip to direct the spin on the ball. Everyday activities can include use of handheld devices such as a cell phone or tablet, in which people grip the device but also use their fingers to access the content. Typing on a laptop or keyboard, with the forearms sitting below the keyboard, forces wrist extension with finger flexion and can be implicated in forearm pain. Occupational athletes, such as those who use manual tools, combine grip strength with forearm strength. Electric tools, while being easier from an isotonic action perspective, produce vibrations that require isometric control of the forearm muscles. Of course, issues above the forearm in the kinetic chain, such as shoulder instability, can place the muscles in a position that causes increased stress.

Lower-Extremity Stressors

The lower extremities are forced to adapt to changes that occur from the ground up. Anything from footwear (or lack thereof) to the type of surface to differences in leg length may or may not cause issues. One of the first and most important rules for treating the lower extremity is not to fix something that is not broken. As a runner, I often hear people encouraging changes such as midfoot striking (as opposed to a heel strike) or zero-drop shoes to improve performance. As discussed in other chapters regarding the research on massage (chapter 3) and on additional self-care therapies (chapter 11), none of these changes are specifically related to performance outcomes. For individuals without injuries, forcing a new type of running can increase their chance of injury. The body is made to work at optimal efficiency, and people will gravitate toward what works for them. For people battling injury, it is okay to advise them to look to some of these other areas to improve their outcomes. Fitting for the correct shoes can do wonders for people struggling with pain when walking or running. After injury or surgery, some individuals may need to adjust their running gait. However, most people are doing just fine.

Running

In terms of the gait cycle, running and walking have a few distinct differences in relation to the contact of the foot with the ground. In walking, humans have a stance phase and a swing phase: One foot is always in contact with the ground, and there is a period where both feet are in contact with the ground. Running features a stance phase, a swing phase, and a float phase: Both feet are never on the ground at the same time, and there is a period where neither foot is in contact with the ground (figure 5.3). Compared with walking, running requires a greater range of motion at all joints of the lower extremity as well as a greater amount of eccentric contraction of the muscles (Nicola and Jewison 2012). When the foot

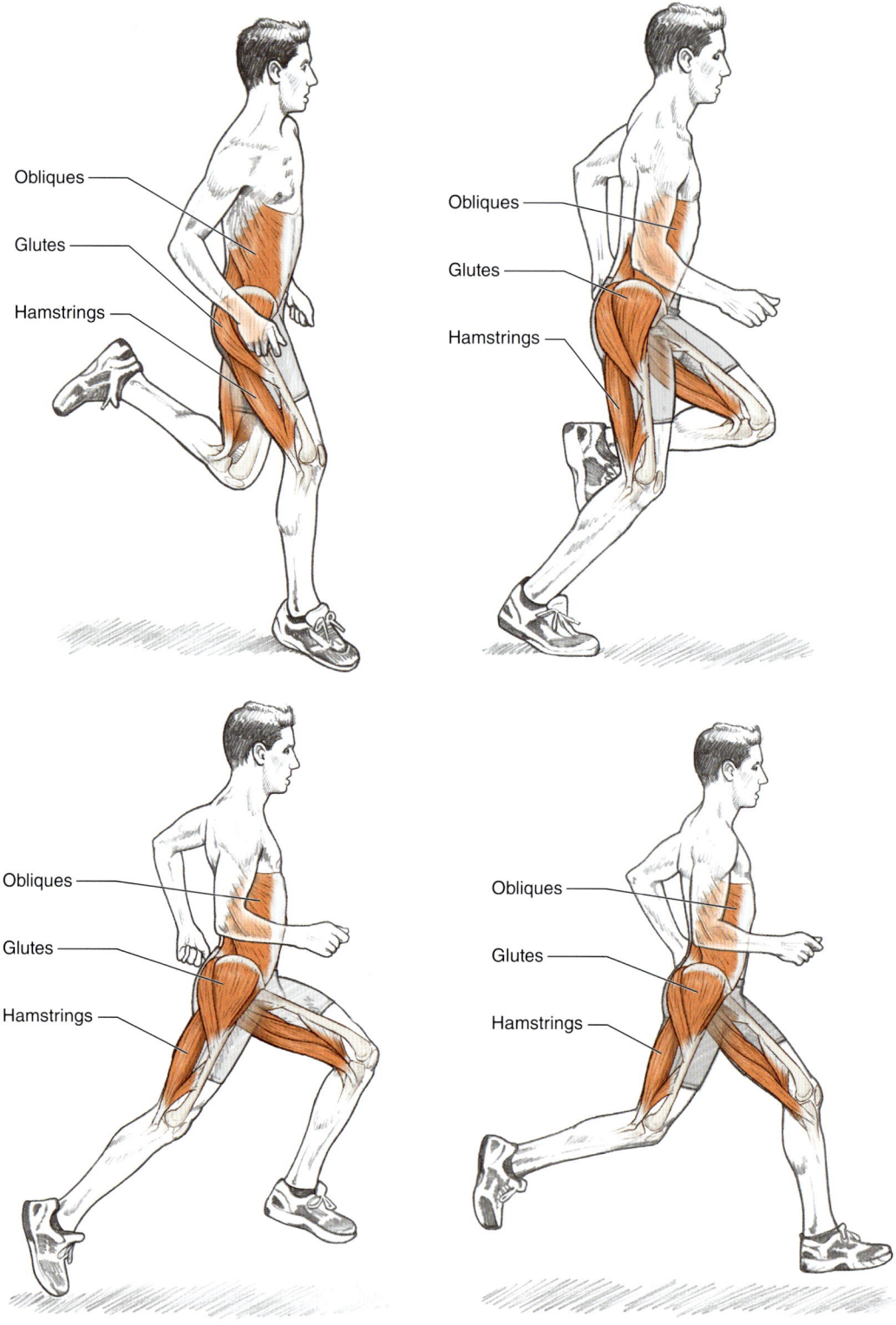

Figure 5.3 The running gait cycle is characterized by only one foot being in contact with the ground at a time and a float phase where neither foot is in contact with the ground.

hits the ground with running, the body will absorb up to three times its weight. The weight is initially absorbed by the foot and ankle before it is transferred up the kinetic chain, potentially influencing the knees, hips, or low back, depending on the person's own unique combination of strength, range of motion, and structural composition.

In terms of how the foot responds to initial contact with the ground, there is a combination of pronation and supination throughout the cycle. Initial pronation of the foot absorbs the impact on landing while helping to maintain balance, adjusting to the surface underneath it during the subphases of stance (Nicola and Jewison 2012). To propel the body forward, the foot moves from pronation into supination. During supination, the position of the tarsal bones creates a more rigid alignment, taking the foot from a supple shock absorber (in pronation) into a rigid lever (in supination) for a more efficient push off the ground (Nicola and Jewison 2012). Pronation and supination are both required for optimal gait. Issues arise when there is excessive motion (e.g., overpronation) or limited motion that does not allow for facilitation between the two.

Movement up the kinetic chain is a coordinated dance between flexion and extension at the knee and hip. Limited knee flexion may lead to hip hiking and excessive abduction to allow the foot to clear. Limited hip flexion may result in increased motion at the pelvis or low back. These adjustments can also be seen down the kinetic chain, where limited knee flexion may force greater dorsiflexion at the ankle and limited hip flexion may result in greater knee extension. To increase understanding of how the body adapts to the stresses of running, clinicians can consult other resources (Nicola and Jewison 2012). Continued understanding of the complexities of the gait cycle is an ongoing process that requires further investigation and skills on the part of the clinician. Even if the clinician does not work specifically with runners, running is an integral part of many other sports.

Cycling

Although cycling does not have the weight-bearing aspect of running, it has its own set of concerns with alignment and posture. The alignment of the bike seat influences the hip's ability to produce force. The distance of the pedal influences the range of motion at the knee. An avid cyclist may clip their bike shoes into the pedals, allowing them to pull the pedal up and push it down (this is different from the bikes used for recreation or from the stationary bikes at a gym, in which the only movement is pushing down on the pedal). Upper-body position during cycling also comes into play based on the handlebar position and the amount of leaning over the handlebars, potentially influencing the upper and lower back.

The bike setup has the largest influence on cycling-related stressors to the body. Body positioning can influence the range of motion in hip flexion because the hip flexor muscles are forced to work from flexion to extension in a more shortened position. Conversely, the hip extensors maintain a lengthened position when in hip flexion but are then expected to engage into hip extension. Wearing shoes that clip into the bike pedals engages the anterior tibialis (ankle dorsiflexor) to pull the pedals up, whereas wearing clipless shoes only engages the plantar flexors (gastrocnemius and soleus) to push the pedals down. The position of the hip and knee in relation to the seat and pedal alignment can affect the iliotibial band and lateral hip musculature. Proper bike setup is outside the clinician's scope; therefore, referral to a specialist for help is encouraged if the therapist suspects positioning might be an issue.

Axial Skeleton (Back and Neck) Stressors

The anatomy of the specific sections of the spine and ribs is outlined in chapters 7 and 8. There is much to consider when examining spinal movement, especially in relation to upper- and lower-extremity movements. As pointed out in the discussion of running and cycling, deficiencies in lower-extremity range of motion can cause the stress to move into the back. Lack of proper motion at the shoulder or misalignment of the scapula can lead to stresses from throwing to be absorbed into the spine. Movements more specific to the spine should also be considered.

The thoracic spine has the greatest ability to produce rotation, based on facet joint alignment. However, if rotation is limited in this area, the force will often move to the lumbar region. Activities such as swinging a golf club, baseball bat, or softball bat rely on rotation of the thoracic spine. If the range of motion is diminished, the force moves to the lumbar spine, which has a more limited range of motion in rotation structurally. Therefore, the muscles will take up more of the force; by placing greater stress on the spine, the person is at greater risk for structural issues, such as disc pathology.

In addition to the transverse plane limitations putting stress on the lumbar region, pelvic positioning also can lead to low back pain. An anterior pelvic tilt with shortened hip flexors and lengthened hip extensors increases the lordotic curve (as outlined in chapter 4). Some athletes, such as football linemen or baseball catchers, spend substantial time in a squat position, resulting in this imbalance. Regardless of whether the imbalance is caused by sport or prolonged sitting (e.g., as would be evident in a race car driver), the treatment is the same. Therefore, the key goal of sports massage is this: Clinicians should know the basic movements and stressor responses in the body and treat accordingly, even if they are not familiar with the sport.

WHY DOES THE CLINICIAN CARE?

Working with athletes involves detailed understanding of how the anatomy responds to the stresses placed on it. Clinicians can always ask patients about the actions they are performing and what is causing their issues. Clinicians should trust their understanding of anatomy, and they should learn the specifics of the client's activity as needed.

PART II

Techniques

The goal of part II is to help clinicians understand the what of developing the treatment plan. Now that clinicians know the why of manual therapy, part II addresses the what by reviewing the anatomy and discussing how to apply the treatments to each muscle. Chapters 6 to 10 are organized by body region for ease of finding the relevant muscles. Each muscle is outlined with its origin, insertion, action, and innervation to serve as a reference. Common stressors and concerns that clinicians may find with the muscle are also described, as done in chapters 4 and 5. Finally, chapter 11 describes self-care options that clinicians can discuss with patients.

Each area in chapters 6 to 10 includes discussion of how to apply the techniques described in chapter 3. However, no set treatment plan for clinicians is provided; this is intentional. The idea is for clinicians to use what they know, what the client on the table tells them (either verbally or through the story their body is telling), and the general concepts of the techniques to move forward. Think of chapters 1 to 5 in part I as ingredients used in creating a recipe. Part II presents options on how to combine the ingredients, but there is no strict recipe to follow. Clinicians have free rein to create the recipe that fits the treatment plan they develop as part of their goals for the session.

Shoulder, Arm, Forearm, and Hand

The upper appendicular skeleton stems from the shoulder down to the fingers. The articulation between the sternum and the clavicle (sternoclavicular joint) is the only attachment for the entire arm to the rest of the body. Movement at all the distal joints relies on positioning of the shoulder and force generated by the arm, and it is dependent on the transfer from the lower extremity and the core. Solving upper-extremity issues can work up or down the kinetic chain, making it necessary to look at all areas.

Most conditions in which manual therapy will be warranted are overuse injuries, although there are some acute injuries for which treatment may be beneficial in the healing stages. Therefore, it may not be necessary to look for a mechanism of injury; rather, it may be more appropriate to examine where athletes experience pain during their mechanics. Upper-extremity sport mechanics are to throwing and racket sports what gait mechanics are to walking and running. Although it is not up to the clinician to change mechanics (that is the job of a coach), assessment may be the best way for the clinician to identify muscles that may be mechanically stressed. Identifying which muscles need to be lengthened and which ones need to be strengthened can help to balance the function of the upper extremity.

Shoulder Complex

The shoulder is a complex arrangement of multiple joints. Three joints—the glenohumeral, sternoclavicular, and acromioclavicular joints—meet the criteria for being a true synovial joint (figure 6.1): the articulation of two bones with connective tissue providing stability in the form of a joint capsule and ligaments. A fourth joint, the scapulothoracic joint, is not a true joint because it involves the positioning of the scapula on the thorax without the assistance of ligaments or a joint capsule. Only the dynamic stability of the axiohumeral muscles functions to keep the scapula in

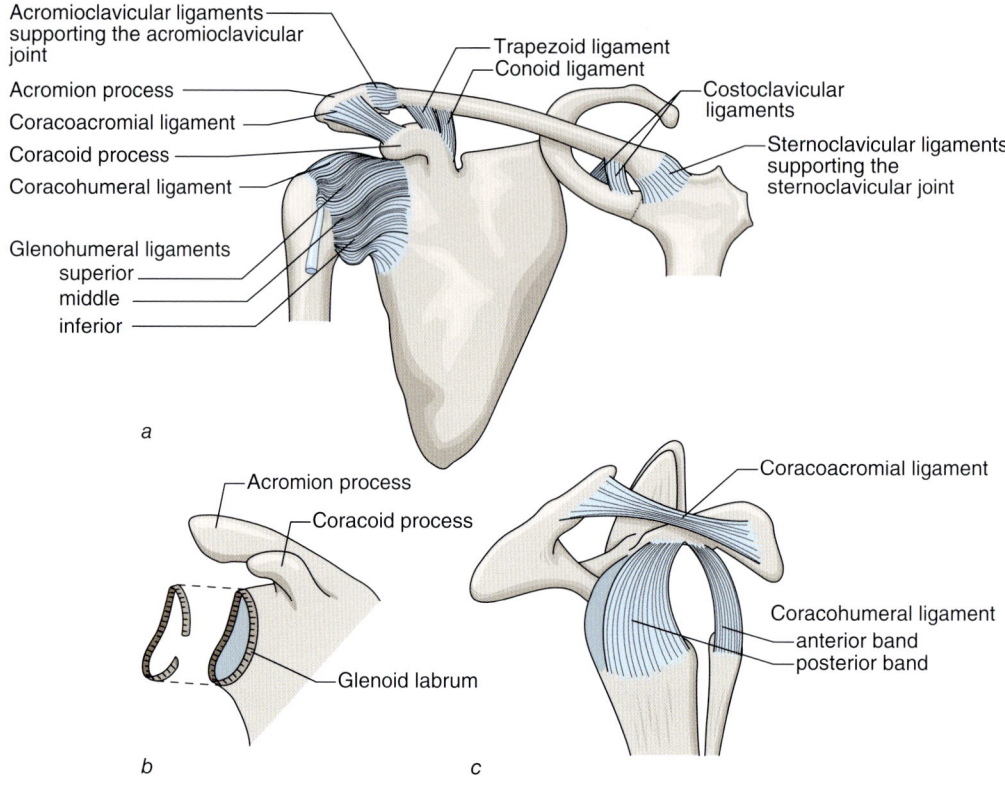

Figure 6.1 The three true joints of the shoulder complex: the glenohumeral joint, the sternoclavicular joint, and the acromioclavicular joint. Although all three are synovial joints, the acromioclavicular joint lacks any actions.

an optimal position to provide the most efficient line of pull for the scapulohumeral muscles (see the Axiohumeral Muscles and the Scapulohumeral Muscles subsections in this chapter). Although each joint of the shoulder complex has its own identity, the synchronicity of the joints provides for effective and efficient movement.

Sternoclavicular Joint

The *sternoclavicular joint* is the articulation of the sternal (proximal) end of the clavicle with the manubrium of the sternum. It is a synovial joint, which can be considered a gliding joint or a ball-and-socket joint (depending on the textbook consulted). The manubrium provides a shallow socket with an articular disc to allow for support of the larger sternal end of the clavicle. The synovial membrane is very strong and is supported by the sternoclavicular, costoclavicular, and interclavicular ligaments. The joint moves in all three planes; however, isolating actions of the sternoclavicular joint without accompanying actions of the glenohumeral joint is not possible. Injury to the sternoclavicular joint is rare, owing to its design (with a strong capsule and ligaments) and the way the upper extremity absorbs forces. Even a direct fall onto the tip of the shoulder is more likely to injure the acromioclavicular joint or cause the clavicle to fracture. However, the number of muscles attaching in and around the clavicle and sternum makes this an area not to be overlooked for manual therapy, even if it is not the cause of concern.

Acromioclavicular Joint

The distal end of the clavicle articulates with the acromion of the scapula (the lateral end of the spine of the scapula) to form the *acromioclavicular joint*. The synovial capsule is reinforced by the acromioclavicular ligaments (between the acromion and the clavicle) as well as the coracoclavicular ligaments (ligaments between the coracoid process on the anterior aspect of the scapula and the clavicle). The coracoclavicular ligaments serve as stabilizers, like cables of a suspension bridge, holding the clavicle and scapula together. When these ligaments are injured, the weight of the upper limb pulls the scapula down, and the clavicle, in turn, appears to move superiorly. The acromioclavicular joint is a gliding joint with no actions occurring directly at it; however, it moves along with the rest of the shoulder structures. Based on its position, the acromioclavicular joint provides a greater range of motion for the *glenohumeral joint* by widening the pectoral girdle. Injuries to the acromioclavicular joint will compromise shoulder range of motion, because the joint involves both the clavicle and scapula and the muscles attaching to both bones.

Glenohumeral Joint

The articulation of the head of the humerus in the glenoid cavity forms the *glenohumeral joint*, which is typically considered the shoulder joint. With this ball-and-socket joint, the head of the humerus balances in the glenoid cavity. The very shallow and small glenoid cavity can only provide bony articulation for approximately one-third of the rather large humeral head. The bony arrangement is best described as a golf ball balancing on a tee. The glenoid labrum serves to increase the surface area of the glenoid cavity and support the head of the humerus; however, injuries to the glenoid labrum are common in people who participate in sports involving overhead motions. The ligaments of the glenohumeral joint blend in with the capsule but are easily stretched, especially if there is a breakdown in the kinetic chain allowing the humeral head to migrate around the glenoid cavity. The rotator cuff muscles surround the head of the humerus for dynamic restraint; because they all originate on the scapula, they can become inefficient if the scapula is malpositioned. The glenohumeral joint freely moves in all three planes of motion (sagittal, frontal, and transverse). However, the overall structure of this joint compromises stability to allow for greater mobility.

SHOULDER LIGAMENTS

The shoulder ligaments are distinct parts of the synovial capsule. The major ligaments include the three glenohumeral ligaments on the internal aspect of the capsule: the superior, middle, and inferior ligaments. The coracohumeral ligament on the superior aspect of the joint, below the acromion, along with the coracoacromial ligament (part of the acromioclavicular joint) provide passive stability preventing superior translation of the head of the humerus. With the positioning of the scapula posterior and superior, there is bony support from the acromion to prevent additional movement of the head of the humerus. The anterior inferior portion of the glenohumeral capsule lacks additional support, making it the weak spot in the joint and the most likely area where the humeral head is subject to dislocation.

GLENOID LABRUM

The *glenoid labrum* serves to deepen the socket formed by the glenoid cavity of the scapula (figure 6.2). Anatomically, there are many variations to the labrum; however, one key component is the insertion of the long head of the biceps brachii into the labrum in conjunction with its bony attachment at the supraglenoid tubercle on the scapula. When the glenoid labrum is torn, the humeral head can move in the glenoid cavity in a dysfunctional pattern, causing alterations to the shoulder mechanics. Although injuries to the labrum are structural and cannot be addressed directly through manual therapy, the residual effects of an injury or surgery related to the labrum may be addressed with manual therapy to the biceps brachii and to the shoulder muscles, which become stressed by the migration of the humeral head.

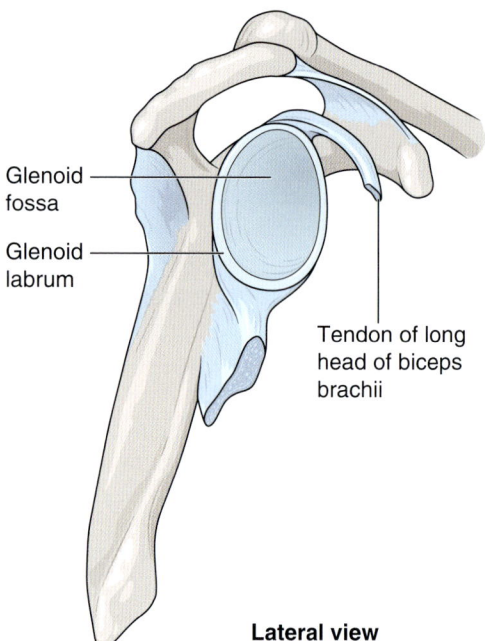

Figure 6.2 The glenoid labrum with the origin tendon of the long head of the biceps brachii.

Scapulothoracic Joint

The positioning of the scapula on the ribs creates the *scapulothoracic joint*. This joint has no ligaments, capsule, or other connective tissue structures as passive restraints to hold the scapula on the ribs. The scapulothoracic joint relies completely on the muscles, specifically those originating on the ribs, clavicle, and sternum, to hold the scapula in place. When any of the muscles are in dysfunction (e.g., postural muscles shorten or phasic muscles lengthen), the position of the scapula is altered from its normal orientation. As the scapula changes its position, the scapulohumeral muscles have an altered alignment. Also, the orientation of the glenoid cavity is changed, thereby changing the positioning of the humerus and affecting the rest of the muscles distally and also potentially damaging the synovial capsule or the labrum of the glenohumeral joint. Although the structural changes to most joints (ligament tears, labral tears, or capsular sprains) cannot be fixed without repairing the injured structures, the muscles surrounding the scapula can be managed with appropriate manual therapy, stretching, and strengthening.

MOVEMENTS

The scapulothoracic joint includes specific actions that describe movements of the scapula as well as the scapulohumeral rhythm. Actions at the scapulothoracic joint include protraction (*abduction*) and retraction (*adduction*), elevation and depression, and upward and downward rotations. Retraction, depression, and downward rotation are all actions that return the scapula to its anatomical position. In addition, when the abduction occurs at the humerus, there is accompanying upward rotation of the scapula, dubbed the *scapulohumeral rhythm*, to allow for the greatest range of motion at the shoulder despite the potential blocks by the skeletal anatomy. Although it is often described as a 2:1 ratio (glenohumeral joint to scapulothoracic joint), the movement through this 180-degree range is more complex. The first 30 degrees of abduction occur just at the glenohumeral joint (0-30 degrees, 30 degrees total by the glenohumeral joint). The next 60 degrees are a 1:1 ratio (30-90 degrees; 30 degrees of additional abduction by the glenohumeral joint and 30 degrees of upward rotation by the scapulothoracic joint). The last 90 degrees are a 2:1 ratio (90-180 degrees; 60 degrees of additional abduction by the glenohumeral joint and 30 degrees of additional upward rotation by the scapulothoracic joint). If the scapula is unable to move in this effective rhythm, either by rotating too soon or not at all, the ability to gain full range of motion of the glenohumeral joint is compromised.

SCAPULA POSITIONING

Normal positioning of the scapula is approximately over the second through seventh ribs. The medial borders should be parallel and approximately 10 centimeters (4 in.) apart, approximately 5 centimeters (2 in.) from the spinous processes of the vertebrae (Moore et al. 2011). The superior angle of the scapula sits about at T2, the root of the spine of the scapula sits about at T3, and the inferior angle is about at T7 (Moore et al. 2011). The inferior angle sits at approximately 10 centimeters (4 in.) from the spinous processes. The normal resting position of the glenoid cavity puts it facing anterior, lateral, and slightly superior (Moore et al. 2011). Deviation of the scapula from its normal position will then alter the glenoid cavity accordingly, thereby altering the position of the head of the humerus. The position of the scapula and the humerus will alter the stress or strain curve on the musculature. By altering the line of pull, the muscle can become less efficient and more prone to trigger points, whereas the fascia can become stressed as the forces shift and tensegrity is altered.

Elbow Joint

The elbow proper, the humeroulnar joint, is the joint created by the humerus and ulna; however, often included because of its location is the joint between the radius and ulna, or the radioulnar joint (figure 6.3). Both joints are uniaxial, with each providing movement in only one plane. Flexion and extension come from the humeroulnar joint, whereas pronation and supination (rotation) come from the radioulnar joint. Each joint is described next.

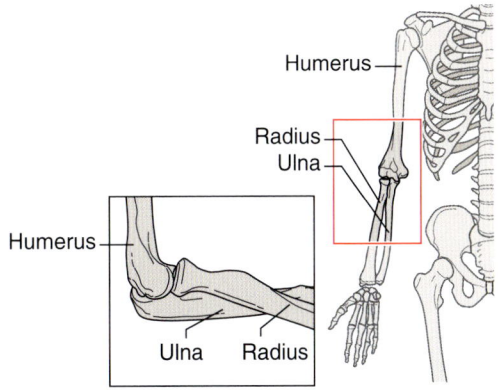

Figure 6.3 The elbow joint is the articulation of the humerus and the ulna while the radioulnar joint is the articulation of the radius and the ulna.

Humeroulnar Joint

The *trochlea* (meaning "spool") of the humerus articulates with the trochlear notch of the ulna, creating a hinge joint referred to as the *humeroulnar joint*. The bony congruency creates a very stable joint with a capsule-and-ligament structure designed to support the joint. Although dislocations are rare, they can occur. Most elbow joint concerns involve tearing of the ulnar collateral ligament. Because of the positioning and influence of the forearm flexors in absorbing force associated with throwing, especially a curveball in baseball, indirect treatment to this muscle group can assist where injury to the ulnar collateral ligament is a concern.

Radioulnar Joint

The articulation of the head of the radius in the ulnar groove creates the proximal *radioulnar joint*, which is a pivot joint where movement occurs when the radius rotates. The actions occurring at this joint are pronation and supination. Holding the radial head in place is the annular ligament, which appears more like a washer surrounding the bone. The radioulnar joint is also a stable joint, with the exception of a condition referred to as *nursemaid's elbow*, in which the radial head slips out of the annular ligament. This condition can occur in young children. Distally, the radius and the ulna also cross each other at the distal radioulnar joint. Pronation and supination at the distal aspect occur with the pull of the interosseous membrane between the two bones as well as the pronator quadratus, more of a dynamic ligament than a muscle.

Wrist and Hand Joints

The wrist and hand are made up of numerous joints, including 8 carpal bones, 5 metacarpal bones, and 14 phalanges, along with the radius and the ulna (figure 6.4). However, most wrist and hand joints are gliding joints allowing for small motion between the bones without extensive actions. Most of the joints with associated actions involve the phalanges, are repetitive from finger to finger, and show

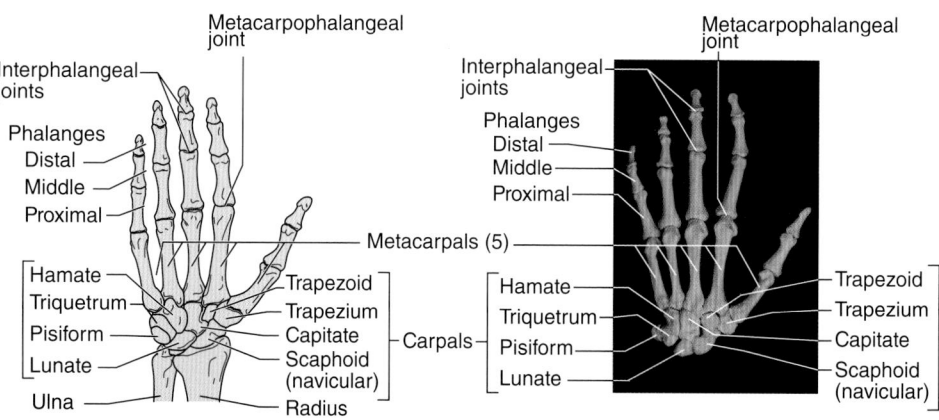

Figure 6.4 The bones of the wrist, hand, and fingers.

a similar pattern as in the foot. The thumb is the biggest exception, which will be explored later in this section. Additionally, there are not many long manual therapy treatments to be done in this area, and the treatments tend to be very specific, potentially putting increased ergonomic stress on the clinician. Therefore, if the clinician works with the wrist and hand extensively, treatment with an instrument-assisted technique would be a better choice than using the clinician's thumbs.

Wrist Joint

The wrist joint proper is the distal end of the *radius* articulating with the proximal row of carpal bones creating a condyloid or ellipsoidal joint. However, the distal row of carpal bones is also involved in the movements of flexion and extension, and the distal *ulna*, along with the triangular fibrocartilage complex, should be considered part of the structure, even if it is not a true part of the joint. Numerous ligaments provide stability to the bones as well as tendons from extrinsic muscles crossing over the joint; however, the main muscle bellies are in the forearm. Actions at the wrist include flexion, extension, radial deviation (abduction), and ulnar deviation (adduction) as well as the biplanar motion of circumduction.

Thumb Joint

The thumb consists of three joints working together to create aggregate motions. The *carpometacarpal joint of the thumb*—the articulation between the base of the first metacarpal and the trapezium—is a saddle joint allowing for flexion, extension, abduction, and adduction, as well as opposition. The *first metacarpophalangeal joint* (the head of the first metacarpal with the base of the first proximal phalange) is a hinge joint, making its actions restricted to flexion and extension, unlike the rest of the metacarpophalangeal joints in the body that are condyloid or ellipsoidal and include movement in the frontal plane. The *interphalangeal joint* (head of the proximal phalange with the base of the distal phalange) is a hinge joint. Also note that the thumb is rotated 90 degrees compared with the rest of the body. For this reason, flexion and extension occur in the frontal plane, whereas abduction and adduction occur in the sagittal plane. The muscles that influence the thumb joint include the extrinsic muscles in the forearm as well as the intrinsic muscles of the thenar eminence.

Hand and Finger Joints

The rest of the joints in the hand and fingers follow a set pattern. The joints between the carpal bones (*intercarpal joints*) and the second through fourth carpometacarpal joints (*distal carpals* with the base of the metacarpal) are all gliding joints, allowing for movement but no actions. The second through fifth *metacarpophalangeal joints* (between the head of the metacarpal and the base of the proximal phalange) are condyloid or ellipsoidal joints allowing for flexion, extension, abduction, adduction, and circumduction. The *interphalangeal joints* are all hinge joints allowing for flexion and extension. Both extrinsic and intrinsic muscles produce movement at the fingers.

MUSCLES THAT ACT ON THE SHOULDER JOINTS

There are four different joints involved with the shoulder, meaning there are multiple ways in which the muscles interact on these joints to create aggregate movements. The complex interaction can make the shoulder confusing, but the key to a successful manual therapy treatment is to keep in mind the function of the muscle and how it responds to stress. Muscles act on either the scapula or the humerus, providing actions at either one joint or the other. Although the muscles that act on the scapula provide scapular movement, they are also responsible for holding the scapula in place to provide a stable base for the muscles going from the scapula to the humerus. Plus, the rotator cuff muscles have the added function of stabilizing the head of the humerus in the glenoid cavity. Knowledge of the muscle locations can help clinicians determine their function, which can help them identify when the muscle is in dysfunction.

Axioscapular Muscles

Axioscapular muscles originate on the axial skeleton (ribs, vertebrae, and sternum) and insert on the scapula. The actions of these muscles are one or more of those of the scapula: protraction, retraction, elevation, depression, upward rotation, or downward rotation. These muscles do not provide movement of the humerus because they do not attach to it. As discussed in chapter 2, any muscle that attaches to the ribs can act as an accessory breathing muscle.

Trapezius

Origin
- Upper trapezius: base of the skull, upper occipital protuberance, and ligamentum nuchae
- Middle trapezius: spinous processes of C7, T1, T2, and T3
- Lower trapezius: spinous processes of T4 through T12

Insertion
- Upper trapezius: posterior aspect of the lateral third of the clavicle
- Middle trapezius: medial border of the acromion process and superior border of the spine of the scapula
- Lower trapezius: base of the spine of the scapula

Action
- Upper trapezius: elevation of the scapula, retraction of the scapula, upward rotation of the scapula, and extension of the cervical spine (bilateral action)

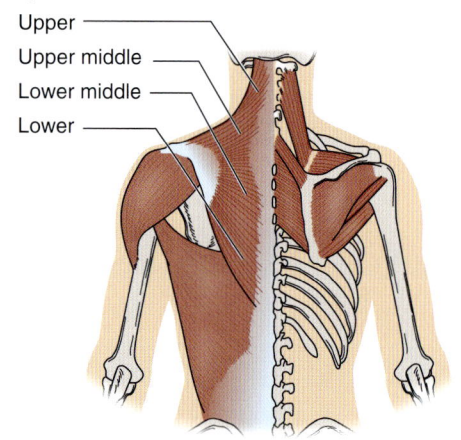

Figure 6.5 The trapezius muscle, named for its shape, has fan-shaped fibers that perform actions at the scapula (all portions) and the neck (upper trapezius only).

Middle trapezius: retraction of the scapula and upward rotation of the scapula

Lower trapezius: depression of the scapula, retraction of the scapula, and upward rotation of the scapula

Innervation

Spinal root of the accessory nerve (cranial nerve XI)

Stressor Considerations

The multiple attachments of the trapezius create multiple lines of pull, resulting in both synergistic and antagonistic actions within the same muscle (figure 6.5). This arrangement results in the trapezius being postural (upper trapezius) and phasic (middle and lower trapezius). Because the muscle features opposing lines of pull and each area responds to stress differently, full treatment requires working the entire muscle where the postural part and the phasic part are treated appropriately as outlined here. The upper trapezius elevates the scapula (as one of its many actions) and is often trained by performing shoulder shrugs with weights. However, because of the postural nature of the upper trapezius, performing this exercise in excess without training the lower trapezius creates an imbalance with the fibers that depress the scapula. When the stronger, shorter upper trapezius elevates the scapula, the scapula is placed in a position that is ineffective for the scapulohumeral muscles. Treatment to reconcile the imbalance involves alleviating the elevation pull of the upper trapezius by releasing the eccentric loading of the lower trapezius to bring the shoulders down. And that is just one aspect of the muscle.

The middle trapezius, like the rest of the scapular retractors, is typically eccentrically lengthened as the stronger scapular protractors and a person's daily activities pull the scapula away from the spine and forward around the ribs. Treatment to release the middle trapezius, combined with stretching of the anterior chest and strengthening of the muscles that perform retraction, will reposition the scapula in a second plane, moving the scapula closer to the origins on the spinous processes of the vertebrae. The synergistic relationship of the three regions of the trapezius in upward rotation relies on the correct position of the scapula to achieve full movement in the range of upward rotation, which corresponds with abduction of the glenohumeral joint. This relationship is essential to the correct ratio of the scapulohumeral rhythm as described earlier.

In addition to its functional considerations, the trapezius is the most superficial of the muscles in the upper back. All treatments of the axioscapular muscles start with treatment of the trapezius. Release of the myofascial restrictions superficially will have a profound effect on the layers below prior to any treatment. This relief will make the treatment seem deeper than just releasing the most superficial layer of muscle. Note that considerations of the trapezius in the cervical region will be addressed with the upper back and neck in chapter 7.

Rhomboids

Origin

Minor: spinous processes of C7 and T1

Major: spinous processes of T2 through T5

Insertion

Medial border of the scapula, at the root of the spine of the scapula (minor), and from below the spine of the scapula to the inferior angle (major)

Action

Retraction of the scapula

Elevation of the scapula

Downward rotation of the scapula

Innervation

Dorsal scapular nerve

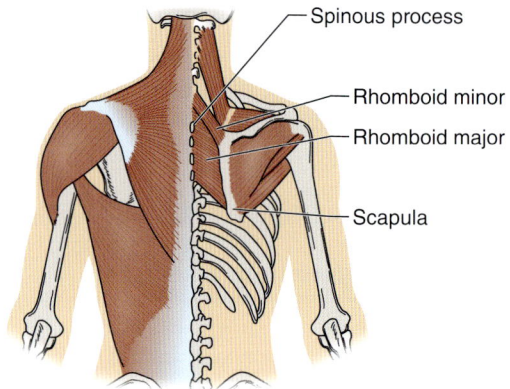

Figure 6.6 The rhomboid major and minor, named for their shape, are phasic muscles that respond to stress by lengthening and weakening.

Stressor Considerations

Although the rhomboid major and the rhomboid minor are two distinct muscles, they work closely together and are difficult to differentiate during cadaveric examination (figure 6.6). Therefore, although the rhomboids are outlined separately, they are considered as one unit in stressor considerations and in treatment. (*Note:* This approach is not followed for all major and minor muscles.) The rhomboids are phasic, responding to stress by eccentrically lengthening and weakening, and they sit deep to the trapezius, mostly the middle trapezius. Because of their insertion on the medial border of the scapula, the muscles are eccentrically strained when the scapulae are protracted. People commonly complain of tightness in this area and feel that they need to stretch the rhomboids to provide relief. However, because the rhomboids are already lengthened, further stretching will not eliminate the issue. Stretching the anterior chest, especially with concentrically contracting the rhomboids by initiating retraction of the scapulae, will relieve the myofascial pain caused by the eccentric lengthening. If the scapulae remain protracted, the body will lay down more connective tissue over time, decreasing the contractility and strength of the rhomboids. Maintaining strength in the rhomboids as well as the correct position of the scapulae will prevent this from happening.

If the anterior muscles remain in a concentrically contracted state and are not lengthened appropriately, it will be difficult to create the correct length-to-tension ratio of the rhomboids. Therefore, as one of my mentors would say, "Lengthen, then strengthen" to create an optimal environment for change.

As noted with the trapezius and what will be a common theme in this chapter, without correct scapular positioning, the scapulohumeral muscles cannot do their job correctly. For example, setting up a strengthening program for the rotator cuff muscles should include strengthening for the rhomboids and lengthening of the protractors. If the scapulae are not positioned correctly, strengthening the rotator cuff muscles will make them strong but they will be inefficient because their line of pull will be compromised. Treatment of the rhomboids will increase the chance of success in treating glenohumeral joint issues.

Levator Scapulae

Origin
   Medial border of the scapula from the superior angle to the spine of the scapula

Insertion
   Transverse processes of C1 through C4

Action
   Elevation of the scapula
   Lateral flexion of the cervical spine

Innervation
   Dorsal scapular and cervical nerves

Stressor Considerations

Any of the stressors that result in elevation of the scapula will affect the levator scapulae. In the case of the shoulder, because the levator scapulae attach to the superior angle of the scapula (figure 6.7), in addition to elevation (its action), the

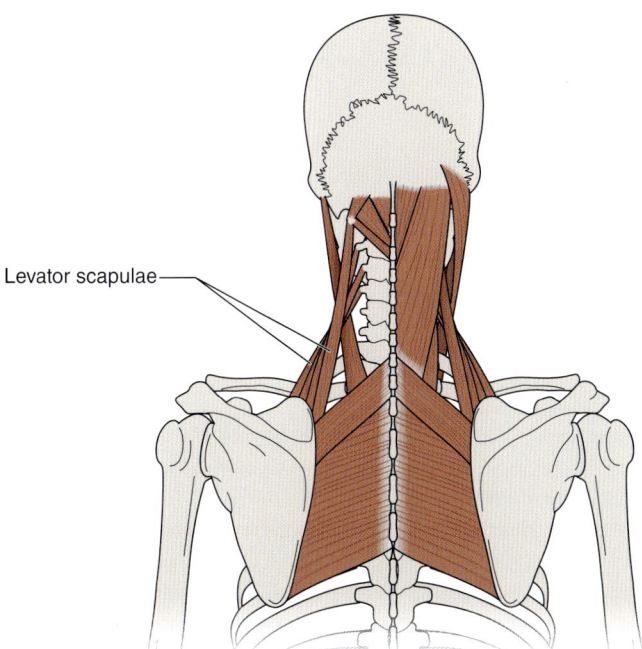

Figure 6.7 The levator scapulae, named for its action of elevation of the scapula, originates on the scapula and inserts on the transverse processes of the cervical vertebrae.

muscle will experience stress when the scapula is upwardly rotated for an extended period of time, even without upward rotation being an action of levator scapulae. Adjustment of the position of the scapula by other muscles will lead it to be shortened secondarily. Palpation and treatment at the superior angle of the scapula may reveal tenderness to the touch, so caution should be used. The levator scapulae is also discussed in chapter 7, because it has stressors in the neck.

Pectoralis Minor

Origin
Anterior surface of the third through fifth ribs

Insertion
Coracoid process of the scapula

Action
Protraction of the scapula

Stabilizes the scapula in concert with other actions (e.g., during upward rotation, it depresses the scapula)

Innervation
Medial pectoral nerve

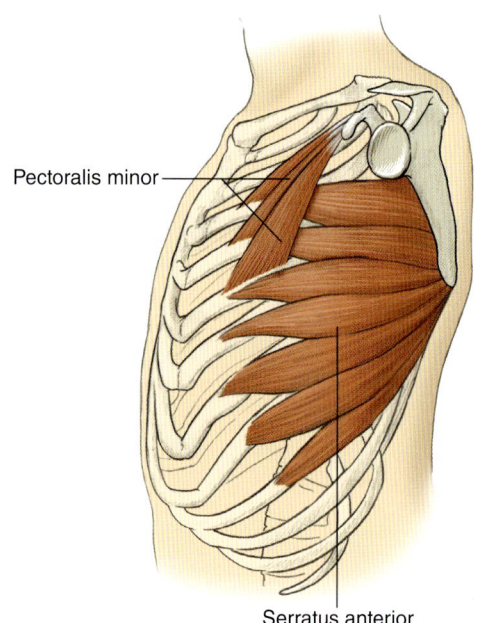

Figure 6.8 The pectoralis minor and serratus anterior are agonists as they protract the scapula. Both originate as slips of muscle on the ribs and insert on the scapula.

Stressor Considerations

The pectoralis minor is a main player in protracted and rounded shoulders. As a postural muscle, it responds to stress by shortening and widening, pulling the scapula into protraction (figure 6.8). Although the result of its pull is normally felt in the eccentrically strained rhomboids, palpation of the pectoralis minor, especially at its attachment on the coracoid process, often reveals a muscle that is tender to the touch. Stretching and lengthening of the pectoralis minor is recommended before strengthening the scapular retractors for optimal results in creating balance.

Because the pectoralis minor originates on the ribs, it also serves as an accessory breathing muscle. Fixing the hands can stabilize the insertion (coracoid process of the scapula) and allow the origin on the ribs to lift toward the scapula. Consider this example of positive use of the pectoralis minor: With the hands fixed on the knees, a person can increase the capacity of the thoracic cavity, allowing the lungs to take in more air. However, with dysfunction of the diaphragm, the pectoralis minor can be forced to take on a more significant role in lifting the ribs to assist in breathing.

The postural response of the muscle to shorten and widen poses another risk of anatomical dysfunction. The brachial plexus, the axillary artery, and the axillary vein pass underneath the pectoralis minor as they pass in a neurovascular bundle from the neck through the axilla to serve the arm. With dysfunction in the pectoralis minor, the person is at greater risk for thoracic outlet syndrome or for other neurovascular symptoms into the arm. Treatment of the pectoralis minor along with the upper back muscles can help relieve symptoms if there is no other structural damage contributing.

Serratus Anterior

Origin
External surface of the upper eight or nine ribs

Insertion
Interior aspect of the medial border of the scapula

Adjacent to the ribs

Action
Protraction

Upward rotation and downward rotation of the scapula; functions to stabilize the medial border of the scapula against the ribs, preventing it from pulling away

Innervation
Long thoracic nerve

Stressor Considerations

The serratus anterior shares stressors with the pectoralis minor as a shoulder protractor and with breathing dysfunctions (figure 6.8). Because of its location, the serratus anterior is susceptible to compression by a protracted scapula. Try this: Place one hand on the lateral aspect of your ribs near the scapula. Now adduct your arm so that the scapula begins to move over your fingers, and begin to walk your fingers posteriorly; your fingers are on the serratus anterior. Clinicians will use this type of palpation to help with treatments of the serratus anterior in the side-lying position, as described in the following sections. Compression of the muscle can further lead to myofascial dysfunction and breathing issues.

In addition to the stressors just described, weakness in the serratus anterior is associated with winging of the scapula. The serratus anterior stabilizes the medial border of the scapula against the ribs. Therefore, if the muscle is weak, the medial border will pull away from the ribs, creating a scapula that looks like a bird wing. Winging of the scapula caused by muscle imbalance or fatigue may not always be apparent; for example, this condition can arise when the person is fatigued and unable to keep the scapula stable. Injuries to the long thoracic nerve could result in permanent winging because the serratus anterior is not receiving the motor response. The long thoracic nerve, unlike most of the nerves, is superficial on the lateral aspect of the thorax, making it susceptible to acute injury but also to damage with surgery, such as mastectomy as part of treatment for breast cancer.

Axiohumeral Muscles

Axiohumeral muscles originate on the axial skeleton (ribs, vertebrae, and sternum) and insert on the humerus. Their actions create movement of the humerus in the glenoid cavity. These muscles anchor the arm to the trunk, and they are involved in multiple movements of the shoulder. For the new student learning anatomy, the axiohumeral muscles can be very confusing because each provides movement in every plane of motion. For me as a clinician, these muscles are some of my favorites because treatment can involve almost every movement and get results.

Pectoralis Major

Origin
   Clavicular head: medial half of the anterior surface of the clavicle
   Sternocostal head: lateral aspect of the sternum, anterior surface of the costal cartilage of the first through sixth ribs, and aponeurosis of the external obliques

Insertion
   Lateral lip of the bicipital (intertubercular) groove of the humerus

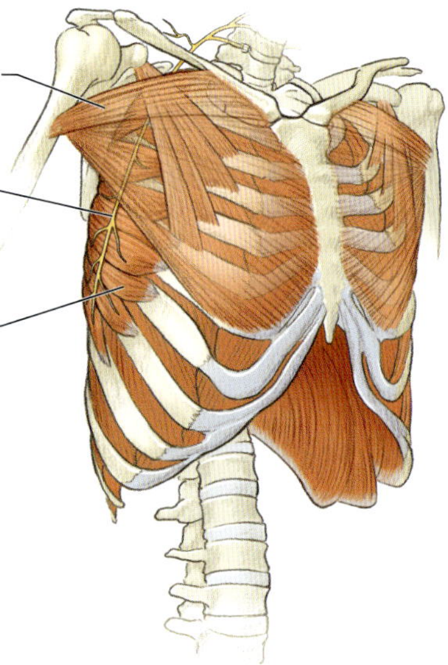

Action
   Both heads: internal rotation and horizontal adduction of the humerus
   Clavicular head: flexion and adduction of the humerus; involved in abduction of the humerus with movement beyond 90 degrees (bringing the arm toward the head)
   Sternocostal head: extension and adduction of the humerus

Innervation
   Lateral and medial pectoral nerves

Figure 6.9 The pectoralis major is an axiohumeral muscle responsible for movement at the shoulder in multiple planes.

Stressor Considerations

The pectoralis major, a postural muscle, is a major contributor to rounded shoulder posture (figure 6.9). It makes up the anterior aspect of the axilla and is technically unable to protract the scapula because it attaches to the clavicle, not the scapula. The broad attachment of the muscle to the clavicle pulls the clavicle anteriorly. Based on the strong attachment of the clavicle to the acromion process of the scapula, the scapula will be pulled into a protracted position by default. It is more appropriate to consider the pectoralis major as contributing to a rounded shoulder posture than to a protracted scapula posture, although the two are not mutually exclusive. The adduction of the humerus at the glenohumeral joint initiates the pull of the clavicle anteriorly, and the postural response of the muscle is to shorten and widen. Additional postural positions related to a shortened pectoralis major include internal rotation of the humerus, a position in which the latissimus dorsi also contributes. Stretching and lengthening of the pectoralis major is the best way to offset its stressors.

Latissimus Dorsi

Origin
Thoracolumbar fascia
Posterior iliac crest
Posterior sacrum
Spinous processes of T6 to T12 and L1 to L5 and slips of the lower three ribs; in some, also attaches to the inferior angle of the scapula

Insertion
Floor of the bicipital (intertubercular) groove of the humerus

Action
Extension
Adduction
Internal rotation and horizontal abduction of the glenohumeral joint

Innervation
Thoracodorsal nerve

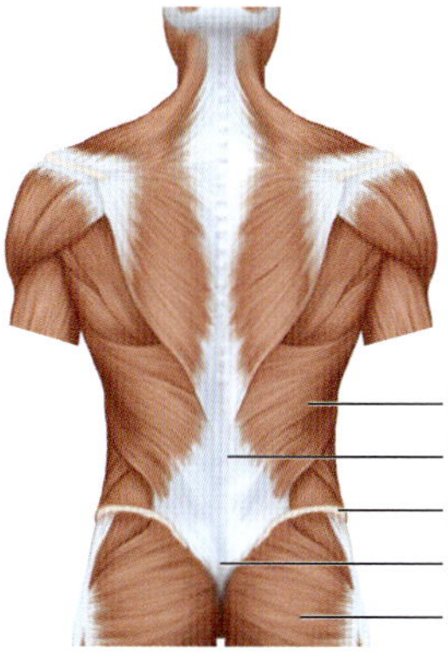

Figure 6.10 The latissimus dorsi, while located in the back, is an axiohumeral shoulder muscle that originates on the thoracolumbar fascia and inserts on the anterior humerus. It also makes up the posterior aspect of the axilla.

Stressor Considerations

The latissimus dorsi is a postural muscle that creates part of the posterior border of the axilla with a tendon that crosses through the axilla to attach onto the humerus from the medial side (figure 6.10). The latissimus dorsi works synergistically with the pectoralis major as an adductor and internal rotator of the glenohumeral joint. This muscle also works as an antagonist to the pectoralis major because it acts in glenohumeral extension and horizontal abduction. The latissimus dorsi is a shoulder muscle although it is located on the back and attaches to the thoracolumbar aponeurosis. Therefore, in addition to stressors at the shoulder, the latissimus dorsi may be a player in low back pain coming from the thoracolumbar aponeurosis. The manual therapy treatment for the thoracolumbar aponeurosis and low back muscles is included in chapter 8 and may be helpful in treating the latissimus dorsi as well. Because the latissimus dorsi also attaches to the ribs, it may be stressed by breathing dysfunction. Based on the location and expansive orientation, the latissimus dorsi is difficult to stretch but does respond well to myofascial treatments such as the lift and shift or the pin and stretch.

Deltoid

Origin
Anterior deltoid: lateral third of the clavicle
Middle deltoid: acromion process
Posterior deltoid: inferior edge of the spine of the scapula

Insertion
All three heads insert into the deltoid tuberosity

Action
Anterior deltoid: flexion, horizontal adduction, internal rotation, and abduction of the humerus
Middle deltoid: abduction of the humerus after approximately 15 degrees of abduction is initiated by the supraspinatus
Posterior deltoid: horizontal abduction, external rotation, and abduction of the humerus

Innervation
Axillary nerve

Stressor Considerations

The deltoid is a multipennate muscle with three heads that act in multiple planes. It shares its origin with the insertion of the trapezius. The deltoid is considered the main abductor of the shoulder, based on its line of pull and the location of its insertion on the humerus (deltoid tubercle) in relation to its origins on the clavicle, acromion, and spine of the scapula. However, the deltoid cannot initiate abduction until the arm is approximately 15 degrees away from the side of the body. Before the deltoid reaches the first 15 degrees of abduction, the supraspinatus initiates abduction. Injury to the supraspinatus (outlined next) can create difficulty for abduction of the humerus by the deltoid.

Scapulohumeral Muscles

Scapulohumeral muscles originate on the scapula and insert on the humerus, acting on the glenohumeral joint. They are not as large as the axiohumeral muscles; therefore, they can be overwhelmed by the other muscles, which also get more notoriety, especially in strength training. The scapulohumeral muscles are often weaker, because they are overlooked via compound exercises and they need more concentrated and specific training than they would get in more complex movements. Trigger points in these muscles will further weaken them (the infraspinatus is my personal minefield). Because the scapulohumeral muscles provide a lot of stability and control for more intricate motions, they should not be overlooked in treatment and should be considered for strengthening as appropriate.

Supraspinatus

Origin
Medial two-thirds of the supraspinous fossa

Insertion
Superior aspect of the greater tubercle of the humerus

Action
Abduction of the humerus, specifically the first 15 degrees lifting the arm away from the torso; functions with the rest of the rotator cuff muscles to stabilize the head of the humerus in the glenoid cavity

Innervation
Suprascapular nerve

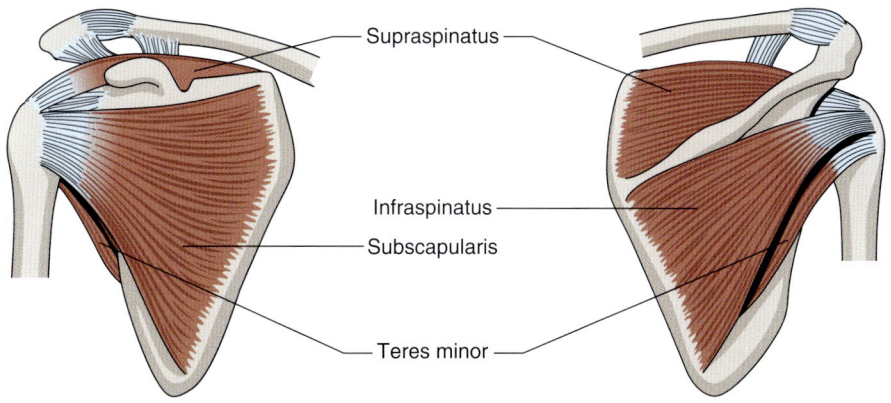

Figure 6.11 The supraspinatus is named for its location, sitting above the spine of the scapula. It is one of the rotator cuff muscles, serving to stabilize the head of the humerus in the glenoid cavity.

Stressor Considerations

The supraspinatus belly sits in the supraspinous fossa, and its tendon runs underneath the acromioclavicular joint before inserting onto the superior aspect of the greater tubercle (figure 6.11). When people view a full skeleton, especially the plastic kind, it looks as though there is a lot of room between the head of the humerus and the acromion; however, in the human body, there is not much space. The available space contains the capsule, ligaments, bursa, and the tendon. If the rotator cuff muscles cannot perform their function of stabilizing the head of the humerus in the glenoid cavity or if the labrum is torn, the humeral head will migrate superiorly during overhead activity, decreasing the space even further. Irritation of the tendon or bursa complicates this migration, causing inflammation and further impeding the already limited space. It is ironic that the inability of the rotator cuff to do its job can continue to compromise one of the rotator cuff tendons even further.

The supraspinatus initiates the first 15 degrees of abduction, lifting the arm away from the side of the body to put the deltoid in position to continue abduction. Injury to the supraspinatus or tendon can lead to the inability to lift the arm away from the side of the body. To compensate, the person will lean the body away, effectively creating the 15 degrees of separation necessary for the deltoid to activate. Dysfunction in the supraspinatus can create a few issues that need to be addressed with appropriate treatment and rehabilitation.

Infraspinatus

Origin
Posterior surface of the scapula below the spine of the scapula in the infraspinous fossa

Insertion
Greater tubercle of the humerus below the supraspinatus tendon

Action
External rotation of the humerus; functions with the rest of the rotator cuff muscles to stabilize the head of the humerus in the glenoid cavity

Innervation
Suprascapular nerve

Stressor Considerations
The infraspinatus is the largest of the external rotators of the humerus; however, it is no match for the large internal rotators, especially the pectoralis major and the latissimus dorsi. Because it is not a fair fight, internal rotation often overtakes external rotation, leading to dysfunction in the infraspinatus. This dysfunction can lead to myofascial trigger points and pain, which further compromises the ability of the infraspinatus to do its job. Treatment can help alleviate dysfunction, allowing for strengthening. Keep in mind the need for the axioscapular muscles to do their job to give the infraspinatus and the rest of the rotator cuff muscles a strong base of support, which they need to function properly.

Teres Minor

Origin
Superior and middle posterior aspect of the lateral border of the scapula

Insertion
Greater tubercle of the humerus below the infraspinatus tendon

Action
External rotation of the humerus; functions with the rest of the rotator cuff muscles to stabilize the head of the humerus in the glenoid cavity

Innervation
    Axillary nerve

Stressor Considerations

The teres minor will often tag along with the infraspinatus, creating similar stressor considerations. Of note are the different innervations between the infraspinatus and teres minor. Therefore, if the motor portion scapular nerve, which innervates the infraspinatus, is damaged but the axillary nerve remains intact, then the teres minor can still perform external rotation of the humerus.

Subscapularis

Origin
    Anterior surface of the scapula in the subscapular fossa

Insertion
    Lesser tubercle of the humerus

Action
    Internal rotation of the humerus; functions with the rest of the rotator cuff muscles to stabilize the head of the humerus in the glenoid cavity

Innervation
    Upper and lower subscapular nerves

Stressor Considerations

The subscapularis is an internal rotator as well as a stabilizer of the head of the humerus. It is not as strong of an internal rotator as the pectoralis major and the latissimus dorsi based on its small size, but it contributes to the motion when the two larger muscles are busy with their other duties (flexion, abduction, extension, etc.). Similar to the rest of the rotator cuff muscles, the subscapularis is unable to do its job if the scapula is not positioned correctly. Additionally, because the subscapularis is positioned on the anterior aspect of the scapula, it lies against the ribs, making it subject to compressive forces based on the position or movement of the scapula. One unique stressor for this muscle is that it becomes compromised when someone is placed in a sling for an extended period. The sustained internal rotation, as well as the lower arm being positioned across the body and the arm being immobilized or limited in its range of motion outside of that position, can lead to myofascial pain and dysfunction. When approved by a physician, treatment for the subscapularis should be done to allow the muscle to function correctly, thereby improving rehabilitation efforts.

Teres Major

Origin
Posterior Inferior third of the lateral border of the scapula

Insertion
Medial lip of the bicipital (intertubercular) groove

Action
Assists the latissimus dorsi in all actions: extension, adduction, internal rotation, and horizontal abduction of the glenohumeral joint

Innervation
Lower subscapular nerve

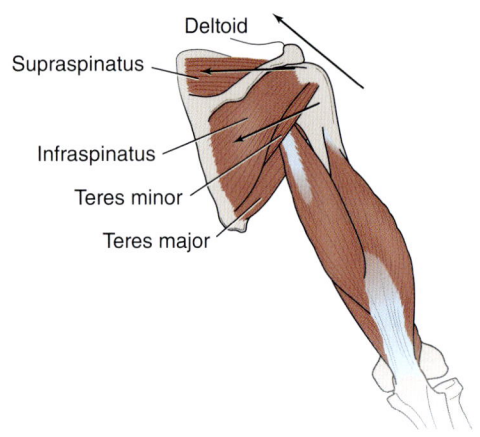

Figure 6.12 The teres major sits below the teres minor on the posterior scapula, passing through the axilla to the anterior aspect of the humerus.

Stressor Considerations

The teres major has similar stressors to the latissimus dorsi because they share the same actions. There are a few exceptions: The teres major does not attach to the ribs or the thoracolumbar fascia, but it does originate on the scapula (figure 6.12). The posterior attachment only being on the scapula places the teres major at risk of dysfunction if the scapula is not held stable. This dysfunction may go unnoticed if the larger, stronger latissimus dorsi is engaged. However, that is not a reason to forget to address the teres major if there is mispositioning of the scapula.

Coracobrachialis

Origin
Coracoid process of the scapula

Insertion
Middle of the medial aspect of the shaft of the humerus

Action
Flexion, adduction, and horizontal adduction of the glenohumeral joint

Innervation
Musculocutaneous nerve

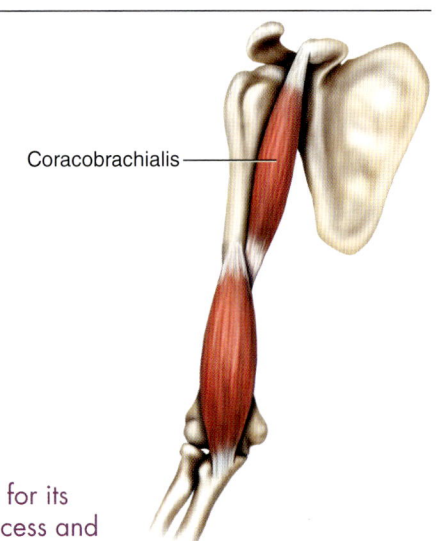

Figure 6.13 The coracobrachialis is named for its attachments, originating on the coracoid process and inserting on the medial aspect of the humerus.

Stressor Considerations

The coracobrachialis inserts on the anterior aspect of the shaft of the upper humerus (figure 6.13). The coracobrachialis alone is not typically implicated in injuries or common stressor dysfunctions, but it should not be ignored. The most common stressor would come secondary to excessive workouts focusing on the chest (bench press and chest flys). The coracobrachialis shares an origin at the coracoid process of the scapula with the pectoralis minor and the short head of the biceps brachii, making that bony landmark an area of tenderness and biomechanical stress. Additionally, the musculocutaneous nerve can be trapped with overuse of the coracobrachialis if the dysfunction is not treated. Because of the potential for concerns at its origin and for the musculocutaneous nerve, it is worth examining this muscle if dysfunction is present in the area. Treatment would not take much additional time and could prevent a more serious issue later.

Anterior Shoulder Treatment

Treatment for the anterior shoulder starts with the patient positioned supine, but it also uses the side-lying position for the clinician to access the muscles. For patients with breast tissue, the techniques described can be used with the patient wearing a tank top or sports bra (depending on their comfort level). This clothing will allow for enough access to the clavicle and superior part of the sternum without being invasive. During the treatment, breast tissue will fall away, either to the sides when the patient is supine or toward the table when they are in a side-lying position, assuming it is natural tissue; augmented breast tissue will remain in place. As the clinician, it is important for you to respect the clothing as a boundary by not working underneath articles of clothing or moving clothing out of the way without the patient's permission. This respect is true for all patients, regardless of sex or gender identity, should they decide to wear a shirt. It is possible to achieve effective treatment while keeping the patient comfortable and respected. Techniques shown include those with a patient in a sports bra for ideas on how to work around the clothing.

With the patient supine, treatment begins with warming the pectoralis major. Loose fist compressions can be used here. If you choose to use the palm of your hand, ensure your fingers are not engaging with or otherwise touching breast tissue or the nipple region. You can position yourself at the top of the table (near the patient's head) or along the side of the table for warming. Remember to use a staggered stance or lunge position. Moving to different positions around the table can help maintain good mechanics as you use the warm-up to examine the tissue for any areas of concern.

Because of the properties of tensegrity, effective treatment of the pectoralis major does not have to involve the entire muscle belly. Treatment can focus on the attachments at the clavicle, upper sternum, and axillary region, allowing the treatment to remain noninvasive. Following the warm-up, fingertip glides can be done just off the clavicle. Position yourself at the top of the table, maintaining a lunge stance. Use your fingertips to traction the pectoralis major from its attachment at the clavicle, starting medially at the sternum, and work a small area until it softens before you move laterally to the next section. Keeping the work to the area just distal to the clavicle will release the clavipectoral fascia without being invasive. The same treatment can be applied to the sternum: Position yourself either at the top of or on the opposite side of the table to traction the tissue off the sternum using your fingertips, working along the areas available on the patient (who is wearing a tank top or sports bra). Depending on the amount of area available, there may only be the opportunity for two or three sets of glides off the sternum.

After the origin of the muscle has been treated, treatment can move to the insertion and the muscle belly along the anterior axilla (figure 6.14a). Position yourself on the side of the table, and use a pincer grip of one or two hands to grasp the muscle in the anterior axillary region, between the humerus and the ribs. Make sure to grasp the entire muscle between your fingers and thumb. From here, use gentle traction to move the muscle linearly from the ribs and from the humerus (avoid lifting the muscle; keep it in the same plane moving toward the humerus or toward the ribs). To add movement to the treatment, shorten the muscle by passively putting the arm into horizontal adduction. From this starting point, the arm can be brought into a variety of positions—flexion, horizontal abduction, abduction, or external rotation—either passively or actively (figure 6.14b).

What makes the pectoralis major difficult to learn as an anatomy student is the number of actions to which it contributes. Yet for this treatment, you, the clinician, cannot go wrong with lengthening the muscle using so many different positions. However, use caution in this position to grasp only muscle, which can be identified through muscle testing. To test a muscle, you want to resist the action of the muscle. With manual therapy treatment, you can use the contraction to confirm that you are grabbing the correct muscle, because you will feel it contract in your hands.

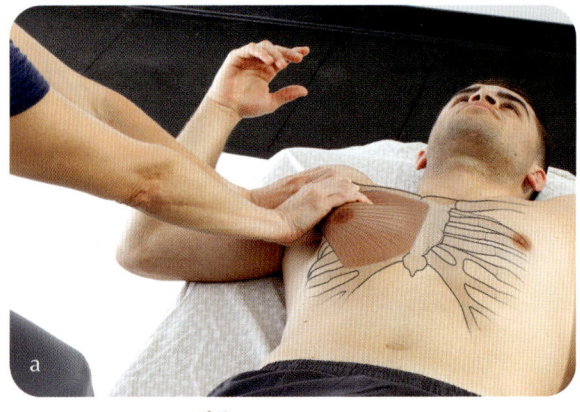
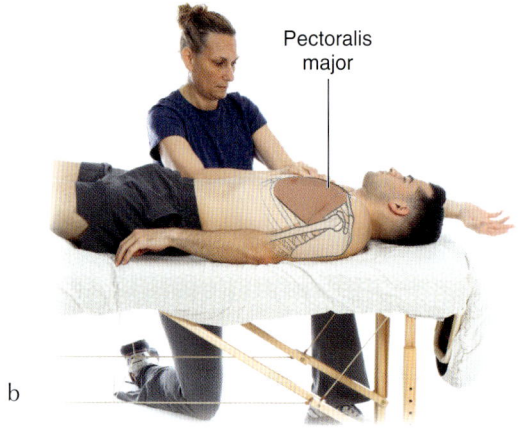

Figure 6.14 (a) Lift and shift treatment of the pectoralis major and (b) pin and stretch treatment of the pectoralis major.

Once the pectoralis major has been treated, the deeper muscles of the pectoralis minor and the serratus anterior can be addressed. For the easiest access to these muscles and the best use of body mechanics, place the patient in a side-lying position (figure 6.15). The patient's legs can be positioned comfortably as long as they can keep their shoulders pointed toward the ceiling, maintaining the position directly on their side. The patient's head can be supported with a pillow. Both arms should be at 90 degrees of shoulder flexion and 90 degrees of elbow flexion, with the bottom hand supporting the top arm. This position opens more space in the axilla to work the scapular protractors, pectoralis minor, and serratus anterior. For the pectoralis minor treatment, stand behind the patient to access the anterior aspect of the ribs with your fingertips. Treatment for the pectoralis minor starts with moving your fingers along the ribs in the direction of the coracoid process until you run into the edge of the pectoralis minor (I refer to it as "hitting a speed bump"). Once you reach the muscle, gently move your fingertips along the muscle with deviation of the wrist. The movement of the fingertips is subtle but effective. Make sure to keep checking in with the patient about how they are feeling with this treatment. Keep in mind that the subtle movement with the fingers will affect the myofascial system overall, especially when combined with stretching and strengthening.

The same side-lying position is used to treat the serratus anterior (figure 6.16). Switch your position on the side of the table so you now are facing the patient. From this position, the fingertips of one hand will rest on the ribs, with glides performed on the ribs headed toward the medial border of the scapula. To enhance the treatment, have the patient put the hand of the arm you are working (the top hand) on your shoulder. As they reach forward, it will open more space between the ribs and scapula, exposing more muscle for you to address. To gain even more space, you can reach the free hand to the medial border of the scapula, mobilizing the scapula to create more space to address. Make sure to slowly disengage from the scapula prior to moving your hands off the ribs.

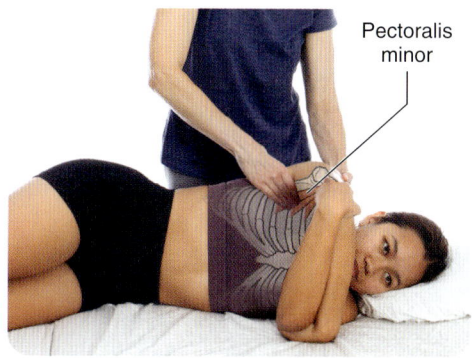

Figure 6.15 Side-lying pectoralis minor treatment on a female patient. This treatment should be done after pectoralis major treatment as it will allow for better mobilization of the deeper pectoralis minor muscle.

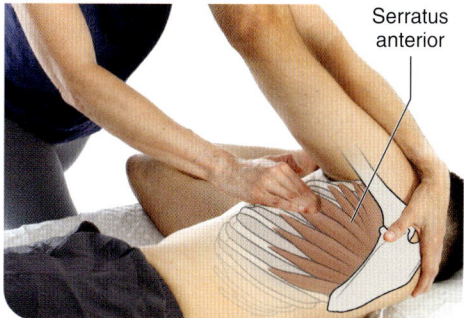

Figure 6.16 Side-lying serratus anterior treatment is performed facing the client with fingertips on the ribs, headed toward the medial border of the scapula.

Posterior Shoulder Treatment

Posterior shoulder treatment, as outlined here, covers the rotator cuff muscles, the teres major, the latissimus dorsi, and the posterior deltoid. The trapezius and the rhomboids are also involved with the posterior shoulder as well as the upper back. The full treatment for the trapezius and the rhomboids is found in chapter 7 and can be used in conjunction with the treatment outlined here as necessary.

Warming of the upper back and posterior shoulders can be done with compressions and some fascial spreading. Face into the table and place your hands on the patient's back, using the heel of the hand or your loose fist. For compressions, you can engage and twist your hand or fist. For fascial spreading to elicit a stretch, lay both of your hands on the patient's back; the hands should be crossed, facing the opposite direction. As you engage in the tissue, create a pull in opposing directions with your hands as the fascia guides your hands apart (do not force this; let the fascia pull your hands). If you are addressing the rotator cuff muscles, include compressions of the muscles on the scapula (infraspinatus, teres major, and teres minor) as well as compression of the scapula on the ribs to warm up the subscapularis. For the latissimus dorsi, include warming in the lower back, down to the iliac crest and the top of the sacrum. This general warm-up does not need to focus on any specific structure, but it provides an opportunity to increase blood flow to warm the tissues. The warm-up can be done to the entire back region before moving to specific treatments of the musculature. The time spent warming and engaging the tissues can also be used for palpation purposes to note any areas of tension or restriction that may not have been obvious from the initial clinician intake and history.

Treatment of the posterior rotator cuff muscles involves glides in the appropriate fossa of the scapula. For the supraspinatus, stand at the top of the table on the opposite side of the muscle you are working while in a lunge position, and use braced thumbs in the supraspinous fossa. Keep in mind that the muscle is deep to the upper trapezius, so you will be working through the layer. For the infraspinatus and the teres minor, the glides are done in the infraspinous fossa, with you positioned either cross table (the same location as for the supraspinatus) or from the same side and using the fingertips or the heel of the hand. In addressing these two muscles, keep in mind that the fiber direction of the muscles is fan shaped from all edges of the infraspinous fossa toward the humerus, with the tendons just under the spine of the scapula. The posterior deltoid can also be treated with glides from the inferior aspect of the spine of the scapula toward the deltoid tuberosity. Movement of the humerus can be added to enhance the treatment for these muscles.

Latissimus dorsi treatments can be done with the client positioned either prone or supine; the prone treatment is described here to start. After warming down to the lumbar region, glides using the heel of the hand or the palm can be done from the inferior angle of the scapula toward the sacrum. Position yourself on the same side of the table, facing the client's feet to work from the humerus to the sacrum. To add movement to the glides, use your inside hand to move the arm into abduction while your outside hand glides toward the sacrum, creating an opposition in pull.

The latissimus dorsi, a flat muscle that makes up the posterior aspect of the axilla, is a good candidate for techniques such as the lift and shift or the pin and stretch.

Chapter 6 Shoulder, Arm, Forearm, and Hand

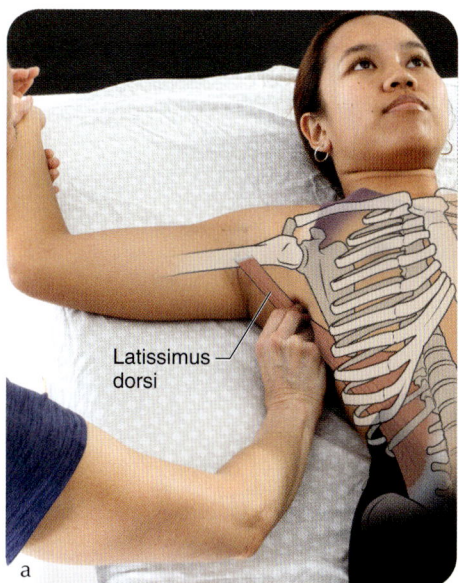

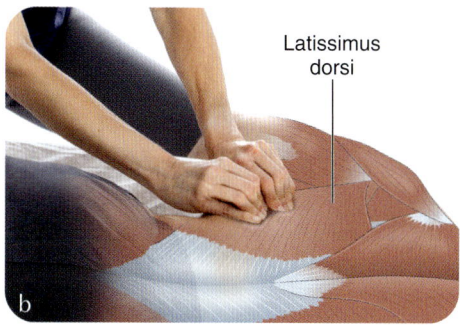

Figure 6.17 Pin and stretch to latissimus dorsi can be performed in the (a) supine or (b) prone position, depending on preference.

For the prone pin and stretch, facing the head of the table, use your inside hand to grasp the muscle belly just at the level of the inferior angle of the scapula (figure 6.17b). Your fingers will be on the top of the muscle, with your thumbs on the bottom. The patient's arm can hang off the side of the table to open the axillary space. Grasping the muscle, lift and shift off the humerus toward the ilium and off the ilium toward the humerus. Adding movement can enhance the stretch, although this requires some finesse. If the patient can assist, have them lift the arm over their head (abduction) while you provide traction toward the ilium. Hold on to the muscle securely when the patient begins to move, because the muscle is likely to pull from your grasp. Make sure the patient's movement is slow and controlled.

Although this treatment concentrates on the latissimus dorsi, it also affects the teres major, which is just off the inferior angle of the scapula. If you wish the address the teres major specifically, muscle test to confirm you are on the muscle belly. Should you wish to treat the latissimus dorsi in the supine position (figure 6.17a), grasp the muscle belly just below the inferior angle of the scapula; have the patient slowly lift their arm over their head in the same plane as the table (not lifting their arm toward the ceiling, but directly overhead). Make sure the muscle is warmed appropriately before the supine treatment by warming the muscle prone.

After the subscapularis is warmed with the patient prone, it is then treated with the patient supine (figure 6.18). Place the patient in the supine position with the arm of the involved side abducted. Face the table; your hand closest to the patient's feet will be used for the treatment, and your hand closest to the patient's head will be used to direct their arm. With the patient's arm in abduction, place the fingertips of your treatment hand on the subscapularis (the nail beds will be against the ribs). Rest your fingertips on the subscapularis. For this treatment, it is not necessary to push your fingers under the scapula; directing the arm will pull the scapula under the fingers (6.18a). Slowly bring the patient's arm from an abducted position to a position where their shoulder is in 90 degrees of flexion. At this point, more of the treating fingers will be hidden, so to speak, between the scapula and the ribs.

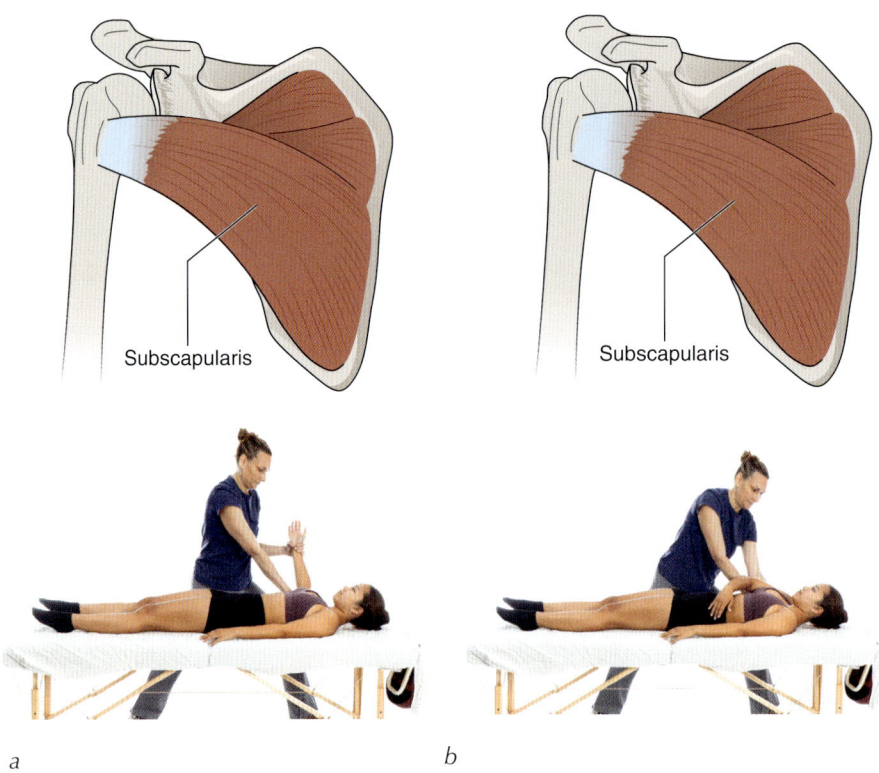

Figure 6.18 *(a)* Start of the subscapularis treatment as the fingertips slowly engage in the muscle; *(b)* the patient can guide the treatment by bringing their arm across their body toward the opposite hip. Make sure to disengage back to the starting treatment position before removing your fingers from the muscle.

From that position, let the patient take control of their arm to control the pressure. Instruct the patient to slowly bring their arm across to the opposite hip as best they can (6.18*b*). If the patient expresses that the pressure is too much, instruct them to back off.

This treatment relies just on the pressure of the fingertips on the muscle, so hang out in this space as long as necessary or comfortable. Exit the treatment the same way you entered: Have the patient slowly bring their arm back to 90 degrees of flexion, then passively move into abduction until your fingertips are cleared from the space. (*Note:* Do not pull your fingers out. Let them be pushed out of the space.) This technique should not be performed multiple times in the same treatment; consider it a one-and-done for the day.

ELBOW AND RADIOULNAR JOINT MUSCLES

Although the elbow and the radioulnar joint are two separate joints with very different functions, they are grouped together for treatment purposes because many of the muscles overlap in location. As learned in chapter 1, the fascia is continuous from area to area, meaning these adjacent muscles may adopt some of the tension from their neighbors with different functions. Additionally, although the biceps brachii and the triceps brachii originate proximally with the shoulder, they are better served with this grouping for treatment and function purposes. Overlap in location also means overlap in treatment, as clinicians may not know if this dysfunction is in the proximal or distal part of the muscle.

Biceps Brachii

Origin
Short head: coracoid process of the scapula
Long head: supraglenoid tubercle of the scapula

Insertion
Both heads converge to insert into the radial tuberosity and the bicipital fascia

Action
Flexion and abduction of the glenohumeral joint (weak in both)
Flexion of the humeroulnar joint (elbow)
Supination of the radioulnar joint

Innervation
Musculocutaneous nerve

Stressor Considerations

Although the actions of the biceps brachii at the shoulder are not as strong as the other muscles crossing the glenohumeral joint, the proximal tendons play a role in dysfunction at the shoulder (figure 6.19). The long head of the biceps brachii originates on the supraglenoid tubercle (a tiny bump on the superior part of the glenoid cavity) and to get there must attach on or around the glenoid labrum. Pull from the tendon may be related to a labral tear, meaning the presence of a labral tear will negatively affect muscle function. In the process of recovery from surgery, the biceps brachii would need to be addressed. In addition, the tendon of the long head sits in the intertubercular (bicipital) groove on its way to the muscle belly. The presence of bicipital tendonitis or bicipital tendon subluxation can also lead to dysfunction in the muscle belly. The tendon from the short head shares its attachment with the pectoralis minor and the coracobrachialis, making it subject to the pull of those muscles. Despite it getting all the attention, the biceps brachii is not the strongest elbow flexor. However, the biceps brachii is the strongest supinator at the radioulnar joint. Because the biceps brachii attaches directly into the radius and indirectly into the ulna via the bicipital fascia, it cannot be as strong in elbow flexion. It also crosses three joints (glenohumeral, humeroulnar, and radioulnar), making it less efficient in elbow flexion than the brachialis, which only crosses the humeroulnar joint. However, dysfunction at the shoulder will continue down the muscle, potentially leading to issues in the muscle bellies.

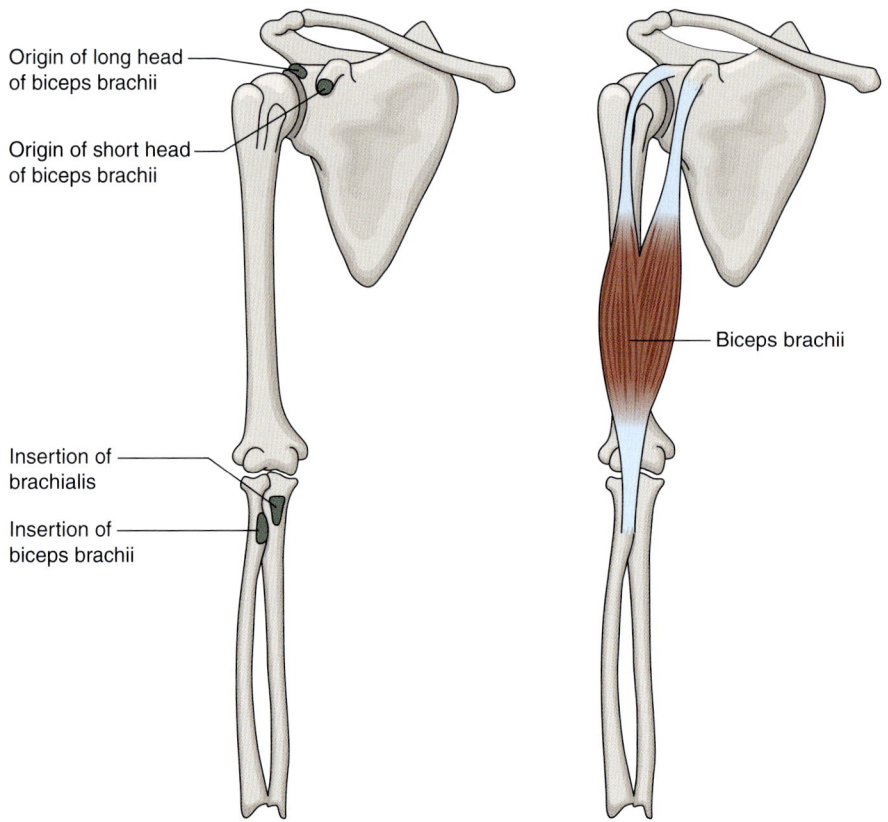

Figure 6.19 The biceps brachii crosses the shoulder, elbow, and radioulnar joints, meaning it acts on all three joints. Despite being known for elbow flexion, it is actually strongest in supination.

Brachialis

Origin
Distal half of the anterior shaft of the humerus

Insertion
Coronoid process of the ulna

Action
Flexion of the humeroulnar joint (elbow)

Innervation
Musculocutaneous nerve

Stressor Considerations

The brachialis is the strongest elbow flexor. It only crosses one joint (humeroulnar joint) and can concentrate all of its efforts on elbow flexion (figure 6.20). The brachialis is deep to the biceps brachii, meaning it needs to be worked either through the muscle belly of or at the sides of the biceps brachii (this is a similar arrangement to that seen with the gastrocnemius and the soleus).

Chapter 6 Shoulder, Arm, Forearm, and Hand

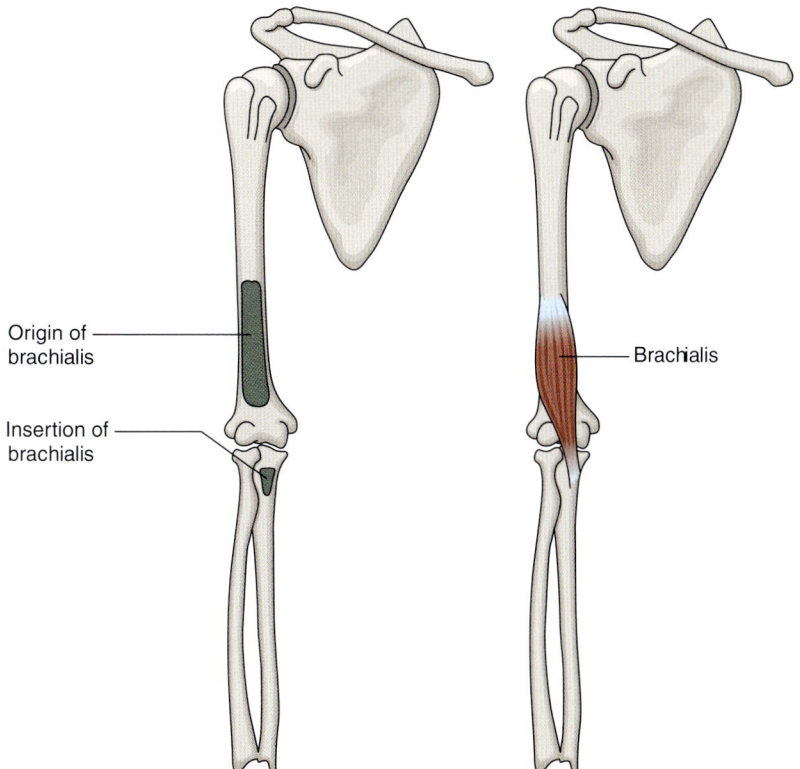

Figure 6.20 The brachialis is deep to the biceps brachii on the anterior aspect of the humerus. While the biceps brachii gets the notoriety, the brachialis is the stronger elbow flexor.

Brachioradialis

Origin
 Distal two-thirds of the lateral supracondylar ridge of the humerus

Insertion
 Lateral surface of the distal end of the radius and the radial styloid process

Action
 Flexion of the humeroulnar joint (elbow), strongest in a position midway between pronation and supination

 Pronation from supination to neutral and supination from pronation to neutral at the radioulnar joint

Innervation
 Radial nerve

Stressor Considerations

Although the brachioradialis is an elbow flexor, it sits very close to the extensor muscle group in the forearm (figure 6.21). As an elbow flexor, the brachioradialis is strongest in a position midway between pronation and supination (imagine holding a drinking glass), performing what are commonly referred to as *hammer curls*. Because of the uniqueness of its location and function, elbow flexion (including an isometric hold of elbow flexion) and any action involving grip strength are stressors of the brachioradialis. The location of the muscle means it will share myofascial connections with the wrist extensors in the forearm. Treatment of the brachioradialis should include the wrist extensors and vice versa.

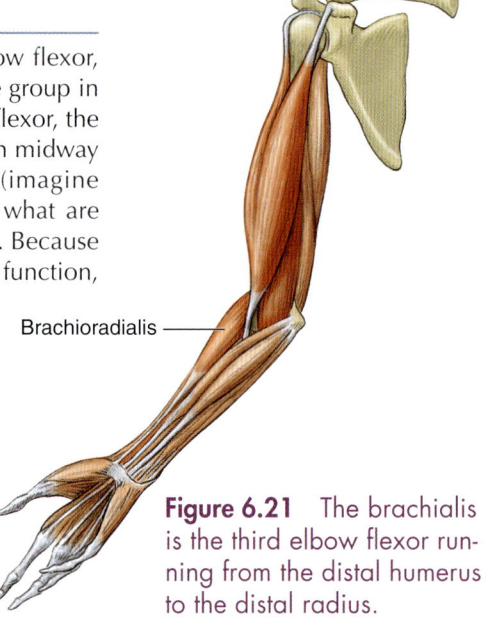

Figure 6.21 The brachialis is the third elbow flexor running from the distal humerus to the distal radius.

Triceps Brachii

Origin
   Long head: infraglenoid tubercle of the scapula
   Lateral head: upper half of the posterior surface of the humerus, lateral to the radial groove
   Medial head: distal two-thirds of the posterior surface of the humerus, medial to the radial groove

Insertion
   Olecranon process of the ulna

Action
   All three heads: Extension of the elbow
   Medial head: is the strongest and serves as the workhorse
   Long head: weak extension of the glenohumeral joint

Innervation
   Radial nerve

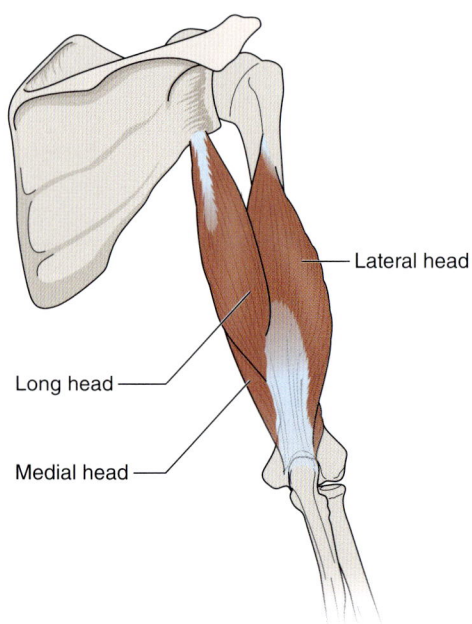

Triceps brachii

Figure 6.22 The triceps brachii, the three-headed muscle on the posterior aspect of the humerus, acts in elbow extension. The medial head serves as the workhorse.

Stressor Considerations

The triceps brachii is a phasic muscle working in opposition to the elbow flexors (figure 6.22). Any activity involving elbow flexion will stress this muscle. The heads of the triceps brachii are named for their location: The long head originates on the infraglenoid tubercle of the scapula, and the medial and lateral heads are named for their position in relation to the radial groove medially and laterally, respectively. The long head, while attaching on the scapula, is not in an effective position to act on the glenohumeral joint because it is below the axis of rotation. The medial head becomes the workhorse in elbow extension, meaning it is recruited first, with the lateral and long heads recruited to assist as needed. Therefore, the medial head is most likely to have myofascial dysfunction.

Supinator

Origin
Lateral epicondyle of the humerus and posterior part of the ulna

Insertion
Lateral surface of the posterior radius below the radial head

Action
Supination of the forearm

Innervation
Deep branch of radial nerve

Stressor Considerations

The supinator wraps itself around the radius and ulna to perform the action of rotating the radius off the ulna to go from pronation (palm down) to supination (palm up) (figure 6.23). Stressors include any action that requires motion between pronation and supination. For example, a softball pitcher who uses subtle wrist motion to create movement on the ball would have the potential to stress this muscle. Based on its deep position, the supinator will be worked with the posterior forearm muscles (extensors).

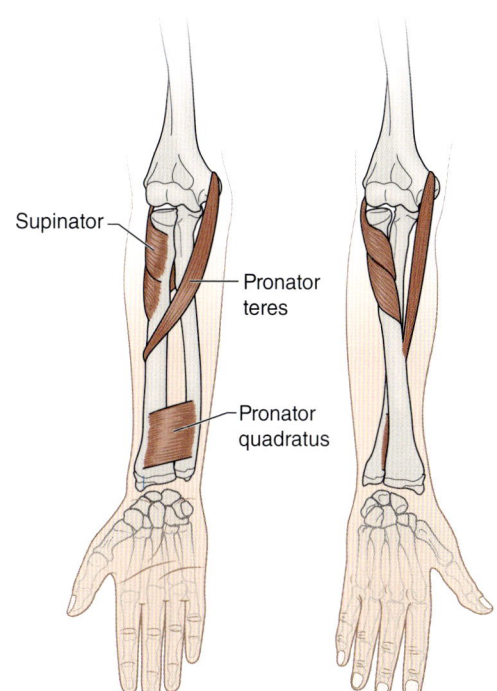

Figure 6.23 The supinator sits on the deep aspect of the posterior forearm and is shown shortened in supination and lengthened in pronation.

Pronator Teres

Origin
Distal part of the medial condylar ridge of the humerus (humeral head)
Medial aspect of the proximal ulna (ulnar head)

Insertion
Medial one-third of the lateral surface of the radius

Action
Pronation of the radioulnar joint

Innervation
Median nerve

Stressor Considerations

The pronator teres is innervated by the median nerve, which passes between the two heads of the muscle. Compression of the median nerve is therefore possible, especially in someone who uses the forearm into pronation, such as with using a screwdriver. Releasing the pronator teres as well as the other muscles in the area can help relieve symptoms from the compression of the nerve. Regular treatments can help to prevent recurrence in someone who is susceptible.

Pronator Quadratus

Origin
Distal one-fourth of the anterior surface of the ulna

Insertion
Distal one-fourth of the anterior aspect of the radius

Action
Pronation of the radioulnar joint; serves as a dynamic ligament stabilizing the distal radioulnar joint

Innervation
Anterior interosseus nerve

Stressor Considerations

The pronator quadratus serves to stabilize the distal radioulnar joint more than it does to provide strength. The muscle fibers sit right along (almost in) the interosseus membrane. When people perform any actions that push the carpal bones up between the radius and ulna, the pronator quadratus, along with the interosseus membrane, helps to maintain the integrity between the two bones. Treatment of this muscle is only effective through the rest of the muscles in the forearm.

Anterior Arm Treatment

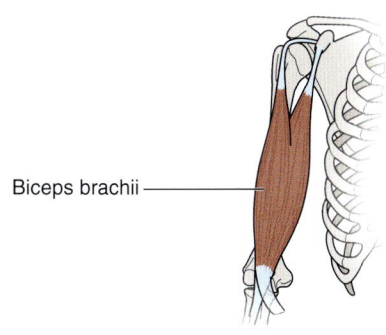

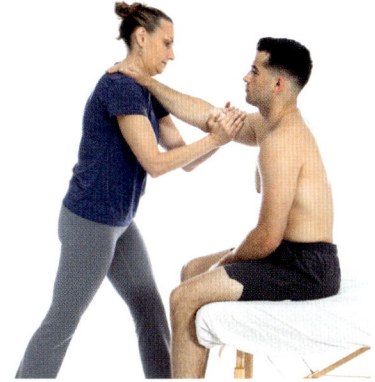

Figure 6.24 Spiraling of the arm done with the arm resting on the shoulder of the clinician.

Warming the arm can begin with spiraling the fascia (this treatment is outlined with the abdomen and thigh as well) (figure 6.24). The patient can be positioned either supine on the table or seated (e.g., if you are working with a baseball player, this treatment can be done seated in a dugout with their arm on your shoulder). Place one of your hands under the patient's arm, reaching around for the most superior and medial aspect of the arm; place your other hand on the most inferior and lateral aspect of the arm. Bring the medial hand inferior and the lateral hand superior, spiraling the soft tissue around the bone. If the patient would like more pressure, have them externally rotate their shoulder by giving this instruction: "Turn your arm toward me" or "Turn your arm toward this hand" (indicating the lateral hand). Because the patient is now in charge of the pressure, they can control the treatment. To end the treatment, have the patient relax first before letting go of the spiral. The spiraling warming technique can be used for both the anterior and posterior aspects of the arm.

Treatment of the biceps brachii is done before treating the deeper brachialis. Treatments can be done with the patient either positioned supine with the arm resting on the table or seated with the arm supported. You can use the heel of your hand or a loose fist to perform glides along the biceps brachii. By positioning the patient's arm in flexion, glides can be done while slowly lengthening the muscle as the elbow goes from flexion to extension. Concentrated glides can be done at the distal attachment of the bicipital fascia. (Treatment of the proximal attachment occurs more with the anterior shoulder treatment.)

The brachialis sits deep to the biceps brachii and can be treated either with glides through the biceps brachii or by working on the lateral and medial aspects of the brachialis (figure 6.25). The edges of the brachialis are accessible on the medial and lateral aspects of the humerus. Muscle testing can be used to identify the location by turning the forearm into pronation and resisting elbow flexion. Glides on the lateral and medial aspects of the brachialis can be done using the thumb to slowly glide from the elbow about halfway up the humerus where the brachialis sits closer to the bone. (This arrangement is similar to that of the gastrocnemius and the soleus.) Motion can be added to the treatment by taking the elbow from flexion into extension.

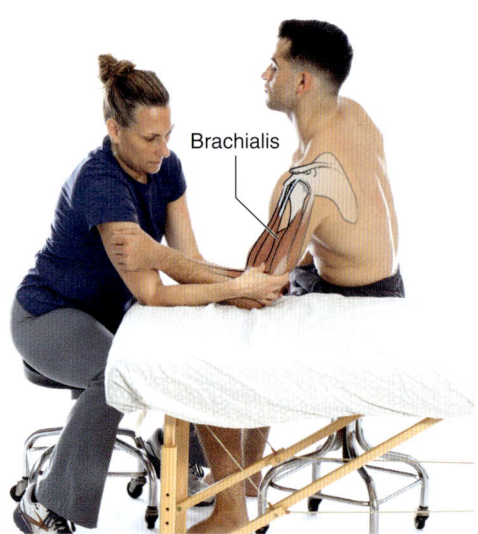

Figure 6.25 Glides performed on the brachialis at either side of the arm to work the muscle deep to the biceps brachii.

Although the coracobrachialis is a shoulder muscle, it can be treated with the rest of the muscles on the humerus based on its location, between the biceps brachii and the triceps brachii on the medial aspect of the humerus, just superior to the brachialis. Glides can be done in one of two positions. If the arm can be slightly abducted to access the medial humerus, glides can be done on the muscle belly. Alternately, the arm can be positioned with the shoulder in 90 degrees of abduction and externally rotated and the elbow flexed to 90 degrees. This position will point the medial aspect of the humerus up toward the ceiling for easy access to the muscle. Glides along the muscle belly toward the coracoid process are an effective treatment.

Posterior Arm Treatment

Treatment of the triceps brachii will mimic that seen with the biceps brachii. Spiraling, done supine or seated, can be used to warm the area before treatment. Positioning to treat the triceps brachii is easiest with the patient prone and the arm hanging off the side of the table. Glides, using either the loose fist or the heel of the hand, are done from the olecranon to the proximal attachment of the humerus. To add motion, start with the elbow in extension and glide while bringing the elbow into flexion.

WRIST AND HAND MUSCLES

The muscles that control the wrist and hand are divided into extrinsic and intrinsic muscles. The extrinsic wrist and finger flexors are on the anterior side (dubbed by one of my former colleagues as the "nonfurry" side), whereas the extrinsic wrist and finger extensors are on the posterior side (dubbed by the colleague as the "furry" side). Any sport involving grip strength can benefit from even maintenance work of these muscles. When treating the extrinsic muscles, it is important to remember activities of daily living that may affect these muscles, such as texting and typing on a computer. The intrinsic muscles are found in the thenar eminence and hypothenar eminence as well as between the metacarpals. Although they are not a focus of our treatment protocol, the intrinsic muscles should be considered as necessary. Detailed information on the origin, insertion, action, and innervation of these muscles is available in a variety of textbooks, including those referenced in this text. Because treatment of the muscles focuses mostly on the area and very little on the individual muscles, they are presented here in groups with the general location given. Necessary information on bony landmarks and areas of interest will be given as needed for creating a successful treatment.

Anterior Forearm (Flexor Side)

The muscles that produce flexion of the wrist on the anterior aspect of the forearm are divided into three layers. In the superficial layer and the middle layer are the longest of the flexors, originating on the medial epicondyle of the humerus. Although these muscles cross the elbow (humeroulnar joint), they are very weak, contributing minimally to elbow flexion. In the superficial layer, there are three muscles. Two muscles, the flexor carpi radialis and the flexor carpi ulnaris, contribute to radial deviation and ulnar deviation, respectively. The third muscle, the palmaris longus, is absent in a percentage of the population, either unilaterally or bilaterally. Presence or absence of the muscle is a fact of genetics and has no bearing on strength or range of motion.

The middle layer consists only of the flexor digitorum superficialis, which flexes only the metacarpophalangeal and proximal interphalangeal joints of the lesser four fingers as well as the wrist. The deep layer consists of the flexor digitorum profundus and the flexor pollicis longus. The flexor digitorum profundus inserts on the distal phalanx of the four lesser fingers, making it responsible for flexion at all of the finger joints. The flexor pollicis longus flexes all of the thumb joints and plays a role in radial deviation and wrist flexion. Keeping in mind the layers of the muscles, where the flexor digitorum profundus is deep and responsible for flexion of all the joints of the fingers, can help make sure the treatment works through the layers if treatment of the finger flexors is the goal.

Common Tendon on Medial Epicondyle

The medial epicondyle is the origin for the muscles in the superficial and middle layers of the anterior forearm. Try this: Place one hand on the medial epicondyle of your opposite humerus, and you should feel the movement of the muscles while you take your wrist through flexion and extension. For me, this used to be an easy way to "cheat" when I could not remember which epicondyle was associated with the wrist flexors and which was associated with the wrist extensors, and it is a trick that I still teach my anatomy students. The tendon of the associated muscles is very short, meaning the musculoskeletal junction is close to the bone. Treatment of the anterior forearm should be angled medially toward this common origin, making sure to end at the medial epicondyle.

Stressor Considerations

The flexor and pronator muscles (pronator teres and pronator quadratus) are found on the anterior side of the forearm. Because more positioning of the forearm is in pronation, the pronator teres is often in a shortened position. The wrist, however, is typically in extension, meaning the tendons of the flexor group are lengthened at the wrist. At the same time, the fingers are often in flexion, meaning the flexor digitorum superficialis and the flexor digitorum profundus are being asked to execute pull at the fingers while being lengthened across the wrist joint. The finger flexors become passively insufficient, which can affect grip strength. For an athlete such as a tennis player, wrist extension and finger flexion are used in forehand; addressing these muscles can help decrease the stress up the kinetic chain where forces may increase at the elbow or shoulder.

Posterior Forearm (Extensor Side)

The muscles that produce wrist extension are found in two layers on the posterior aspect of the forearm. The common tendon of the extensors is found on the lateral epicondyle with muscles originating superiorly on the lateral supracondylar ridge. The brachioradialis, although not part of the extensor group, covers the lateral aspect of the forearm; therefore, treatment in that area needs to work through or around the brachioradialis. Like the wrist flexors, the wrist extensors are weak in actions at the elbow (in this case, extension of the elbow). The superficial layer includes the extensor carpi radialis longus and the extensor carpi radialis brevis, which also produce radial deviation of the forearm, and the extensor carpi ulnaris, which acts in wrist extension and ulnar deviation. Although the extensor carpi ulnaris is a synergist to the extensor carpi radialis longus and the extensor carpi radialis brevis in wrist extension, it is an antagonist to those two muscles in ulnar deviation, where it is a synergist to the flexor carpi ulnaris. Only one extensor digitorum is responsible for extension of the metacarpophalangeal, proximal interphalangeal, and distal interphalangeal joints of the four lesser fingers. In addition, the fifth finger has its own muscle for independent extension at the metacarpophalangeal and interphalangeal joints: the extensor digit minimi, which is adjacent to the extensor digitorum. The deep layer of extensor muscles includes the muscles that extend and abduct the thumb and provide independent extension to the second finger. Extension of the carpometacarpal and metacarpophalangeal joints of the thumb comes from the extensor pollicis brevis, whereas the extensor pollicis longus extends the interphalangeal joint as well as the other two. The abductor pollicis longus abducts the thumb at the carpometacarpal joint and extends the carpometacarpal joint. The extensor indicis provides extension only at the second metacarpophalangeal joint. Palpation of the forearm when the fingers and thumb are moving can help to identify where the muscles are located, even though the treatment will be the same for both layers.

Common Tendon on the Lateral Epicondyle

The extensor muscles angle toward the lateral epicondyle, with the extensor carpi radialis longus originating above the condyle on the lateral supracondylar ridge, along with the brachioradialis. As seen with the flexors, the musculotendinous junction is close to the bone. Muscles attaching to the epicondyle include the extensor capri radialis brevis, the extensor carpi ulnaris, the extensor digitorum, and the extensor digiti minimi. To confirm the location of the muscles, palpation of the epicondyle with active extension of the wrist points the clinician in the right direction.

Stressor Considerations

In direct opposition to the anterior forearm, the posterior forearm has the wrist extensors and the supinator, as well as the brachioradialis, as described earlier. As people tend to spend time in pronation, the supinator is lengthened. With time spent in wrist extension, the wrist extensors are shortened; however, the finger extensors are lengthened as the fingers are in flexion. People also put increased stress on their wrist extensors for activities such as push-ups or bench press, in which the upper extremity absorbs substantial body weight with the wrist in extension. For clinicians performing manual therapy, it can be important to maintain a neutral wrist, especially if they have wrist pain. Keeping a neutral wrist can help alleviate pain in the extensor group.

Hand

The hand features intrinsic muscles that move the digits. Although the hand and the foot have many similarities, the hand features an opposable thumb, allowing people to grasp and use tools, whereas the foot is responsible for gait. Movement of the digits in the frontal plane (adduction and adduction) is considered relative to the midline of the hand, the third or middle finger. In abduction, the fingers move away from the middle finger; in adduction, the digits move toward the middle finger. The muscles that control the thumb are in the fleshy portion of the thumb side of the hand, termed the *thenar eminence*. The muscles that control the fifth digit are in the fleshy portion termed the *hypothenar eminence*. Like the foot, the hand also has muscles that are between the metacarpals and attached to the tendons of the extrinsic muscles.

Thenar Eminence

The thenar eminence contains the intrinsic muscles that control the movement of the thumb. The muscles are nicely named for their actions: From superficial to deep, they are the abductor pollicis brevis, the flexor pollicis brevis, and the opponens pollicis. Medial to the hypothenar eminence in the fleshy portion between the thumb and the second (index) finger are the two heads of the adductor pollicis: the transverse and oblique heads.

Hypothenar Eminence

The hypothenar eminence contains the intrinsic muscles that control the movement of the fifth finger (digiti minimi). Named for their actions, from lateral to medial, these muscles are the abductor digiti minimi, the flexor digiti minimi, and the opponens digiti minimi. Adduction of the fifth finger is initiated by the palmar interossei.

Other Muscles of the Hand

The muscles responsible for intrinsic motion of the other digits are found between the metacarpals. The palmar interossei are adductors of the metacarpophalangeal joints, found between the metacarpals on the palmar surface. The dorsal interossei are abductors, found on the dorsal surface between the metacarpals. The lumbricals originate with the flexor digitorum profundus tendon and insert into the extensor expansion, functioning in flexion of the metacarpophalangeal joints and extension of the interphalangeal joints.

Anterior Forearm Treatment (Flexor Side)

The anterior forearm treatment addresses the wrist and finger flexors as well as the pronator muscles. Treatment can be done with the patient seated, with their forearm resting on the table, palm side up, and their hand near or slightly off the table edge to allow for movement from flexion to extension. To warm the area, start with glides, either with a loose fist or heel of the hand. Make sure to angle the glides to the medial epicondyle of the humerus where the tendons of multiple muscles originate (figure 6.26). You can add movement to the treatment by starting with the wrist in flexion and slowly bringing the wrist into extension. To specifically treat the pronators, add movement from pronation to supination while gliding. Additionally, instead of having the forearm resting on the table, have the patient rest their elbow on the table, flexed to approximately 90 degrees. From here, place your thumb along the pronator teres and slowly pronate the client's forearm into your thumb to create the pressure of the treatment. If less pressure is desired, decrease the amount of pronation of the patient's forearm (return to supination).

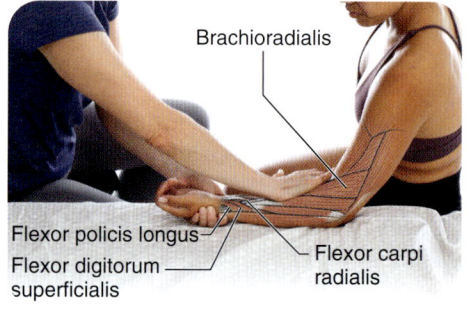

Figure 6.26 Treatment to the anterior surface of the forearm where glides are provided.

Chapter 6 Shoulder, Arm, Forearm, and Hand

Posterior Forearm Treatment (Extensor Side)

Treatment of the posterior forearm mimics that of the anterior forearm. In the same seated position, have the patient pronate their forearm so the palm is down and the extensor or posterior aspect of the forearm is exposed. The hand should also be off the table. Glides on this side of the forearm should angle to the lateral epicondyle of the humerus (figure 6.27a). You can add movement of the wrist, from extension to flexion, during the glides. To address the supinator, gently add supination to the glides. Alternately, position the patient with their elbow resting on the table, flexed to approximately 90 degrees (figure 6.27b). From here, place your thumb along the supinator (aim to place the thumb between the ulna and the radius to address the fascial attachment on the interosseus membrane). Gently supinate the forearm into the thumb to create pressure for the treatment. If the pressure is too much, decrease the amount of supination (pronate the forearm).

You can perform both the anterior and posterior treatments just described on yourself when you experience soreness in your forearms.

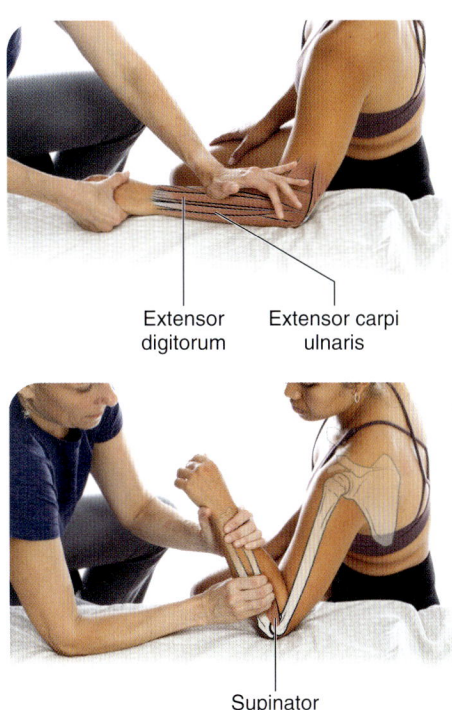

Figure 6.27 (a) Treatment on the posterior aspect of the forearm for the extensor muscles includes glides toward the lateral epicondyle and (b) treatment of the deep supinator with rotation of the forearm providing the pressure.

Hand Treatment

Treatment for the hand can be done in the seated position, especially if paired with the forearm treatments just described. For the palmar surface of the hand, thumb glides should be used on the thenar eminence, the hypothenar eminence, and the adductor pollicis located between the thumb and the index finger. On the dorsal surface of the hand, glides can be done on and between the metacarpals.

WHY DOES THE CLINICIAN CARE?

The shoulder joint is highly mobile, relying on the myofascial structures to keep the joint in the correct position to maintain its integrity. From the muscles keeping the scapula positioned correctly to the rotator cuff muscles keeping the head of the humerus in correct orientation in the glenoid cavity, the muscles of the shoulder joint work hard. Continuing down the kinetic chain, the muscles in the forearm also work with the hand, moving the fingers and providing grip strength. Manual therapy can help keep these muscles in good working order.

Upper Back and Neck

From a sports perspective, the upper back and neck have a few different areas of concern, as addressed in this chapter. Some of the musculature, including the trapezius and levator scapulae, cross over with the shoulder and may be impacted there. Other muscles, such as the scalene group and the sternocleidomastoid, may be influenced more by daily habits of neck flexion. The suboccipital group can be influenced by postural habits, but these muscles can also be stressed from the mechanism of a concussion or even a sleeping position. Some people carry stress in their neck and shoulders, whereas others may hold tension in their upper back while running. Both situations lead to stressed musculature that may not be directly related to sport but needs to be considered for manual therapy treatment purposes.

Cervical Spine Structure

The cervical spine comprises seven vertebrae (C1-C7). The last five (C3-C7) are typical vertebrae, whereas C1 and C2 have some different features. C1, dubbed the *atlas* because it holds up the head (world), is more of a ring of bone, whereas C2, the *axis*, has an enlarged dens or odontoid process on which C1 pivots. The *atlantooccipital joint* between C1 and the occiput (the inferior aspect of the cranium) is a hinge joint, allowing for flexion and extension only. It is sometimes dubbed the "yes joint" because it allows the head to nod "yes." I also refer to it as the "bobble-head joint" because it reminds me of the movement of a bobble-head doll. The *atlantoaxial joint* between C1 and C2 is a pivot joint, allowing for rotation. It is dubbed the "no joint" because it allows only for shaking the head "no."

The rest of the cervical spine is a series of gliding joints where the aggregate movement creates the actions of flexion, extension, rotation, and lateral flexion. Movement depends on how much each vertebra can move on the segments above and below. Rotation, aside from the atlantoaxial joint, is limited in this region.

Thoracic Spine Structure

The thoracic spine is made up of 12 vertebrae that each articulate with one pair of ribs. The thoracic vertebrae feature spinous processes that are longer and point inferiorly, which (along with the ribs being attached) limits flexion and extension; the presence of the ribs also limits lateral flexion. The action with the largest range of motion in the thoracic region is rotation. It is important to remember that rotation has a large range of motion in the thoracic region because if rotation becomes limited, the force is often taken up by the lumbar region (discussed further in chapter 8).

Ribs and Thorax Structure

There are 12 pairs of ribs, with each pair attaching to at least one thoracic vertebra. There are seven pairs of true ribs (ribs 1-7), which attach directly to the sternum. Ribs 8, 9, and 10 are false ribs, which attach to rib 7 and then to the sternum via the costal cartilage. Ribs 11 and 12 are floating (and false) ribs, which do not attach to the sternum. All ribs serve as an attachment for muscles and function to protect the heart and lungs. The scapulae also rest on the ribs.

MUSCLES OF THE UPPER BACK AND NECK

This section starts with the upper back, revisiting earlier discussion of the posterior axioscapular muscles (chapter 6) while adding muscles along the posterior ribs and thorax as well as the posterior cervical region. These muscles are described here because while they are an important part of the shoulder complex, they are also culprits in upper back and neck pain. For example, this chapter revisits upper cross syndrome (chapter 4) so clinicians can see how these muscles are implicated. Although this book can be read cover to cover, the idea behind also discussing the muscles here is to help clinicians create a manual therapy treatment that flows without needing to navigate multiple chapters. When clinicians refer to this book later, they can easily find the information needed depending on the area indicated for treatment.

Axioscapular Muscles

The three axioscapular muscles were discussed in chapter 6, so they are reviewed briefly here. Specifically, for the trapezius, the upper trapezius extends into the neck and is involved in extension and lateral flexion of the neck as well as scapular elevation. The levator scapulae is also a common cause of neck pain, with its role in lateral flexion and scapular elevation. Finally, a significant portion of upper back pain comes from the rhomboids being eccentrically strained with scapular protraction.

As the most superficial muscle in the upper back, it is essential for the clinician to warm through the trapezius to treat the underlying muscles, including the rhomboids. In addition, complaints of pain in this area may not accompany shoulder dysfunction but could lead to said dysfunction depending on the sport.

Trapezius

Origin
  Upper trapezius: base of the skull, upper occipital protuberance, and ligamentum nuchae
  Middle trapezius: spinous processes of C7, T1, T2, and T3
  Lower trapezius: spinous processes of T4 through T12

Insertion
  Upper trapezius: posterior aspect of the lateral third of the clavicle
  Middle trapezius: medial border of the acromion process and superior border of the spine of the scapula
  Lower trapezius: base of the spine of the scapula

Action
  Upper trapezius: elevation of the scapula, retraction of the scapula, upward rotation of the scapula, and extension of the cervical spine (bilateral action)
  Middle trapezius: retraction of the scapula and upward rotation of the scapula

Lower trapezius: depression of the scapula, retraction of the scapula, and upward rotation of the scapula

Innervation
Spinal root of the accessory nerve (cranial nerve XI)

Stressor Considerations

The trapezius remains the most superficial layer in the neck, as it does in the upper back. The upper trapezius is responsible for extension of the cervical spine, but the elevation of the scapula will also assist in creating tension in the neck. Activities done with the head down lead to eccentric loading of all the cervical extensors. In addition, adopting a forward head posture (i.e., leading with the head) can also put stress on these muscles. For example, forward head posture affects the trapezius at all levels, shortening the upper trapezius and levator scapulae and lengthening the lower trapezius.

Because the trapezius originates at the base of the skull, myofascial pain may contribute to headaches and result in tension in the upper aspect of the shoulders. Working through the upper trapezius at the neck and shoulders will allow release of the deeper layers of the myofascial system. Treatment for the trapezius is one of the most used for the upper back, neck, and shoulder on its own and as a start to address issues in the deeper musculature of this area. Note that considerations for the trapezius specific to its axioscapular movements are found in chapter 6.

Rhomboids

Origin
Minor: spinous processes of C7 and T1
Major: spinous processes of T2 through T5

Insertion
Medial border of the scapula, at the root of the spine of the scapula (minor), and from below the spine of the scapula to the inferior angle (major)

Action
Retraction of the scapula
Elevation of the scapula
Downward rotation of the scapula

Innervation
Dorsal scapular nerve

Stressor Considerations

The rhomboids do not serve any function at the neck, but they are often associated more with upper back pain than with shoulder pain. Because upper back pain comes from the rhomboids being eccentrically strained with scapulae protraction, shoulder positioning, as well as that of the neck and upper portion of the back, must be examined. When clinicians look to address a forward head posture, the rhomboids are usually associated with protracted shoulders in upper cross syndrome (see chapter 4). Therefore, when completing a protocol for the posterior neck, treatment of the upper back should be considered. As clinicians aim to return the head to a neutral position to counteract the stresses of forward head posture, releasing the rhomboids will help adjust the superior structures.

Levator Scapulae

Origin
Medial border of the scapula from the superior angle to the spine of the scapula

Insertion
Transverse processes of C1 through C4

Action
Elevation of the scapula

Lateral flexion of the cervical spine

Innervation
Dorsal scapular and cervical nerves

Stressor Considerations
When clinicians look at the actions of the levator scapulae from an anatomy perspective, they see elevation of the scapula and lateral flexion. However, when they consider these actions from a functional perspective, any action in which the shoulder is elevated and the neck is laterally flexed to the same side (e.g., when the ear is brought to the shoulder) will be a stressor to the levator scapulae. For those old enough to remember using a phone without earbuds or a speakerphone, a well-known example of a stressor for the levator scapulae involves putting the phone on the shoulder and bringing the shoulder to meet the ear and the ear to meet the shoulder. Other activities that serve as stressors include carrying a heavy bag on the shoulder or tilting the head to the same side to adjust the center of gravity. Forward head posture and upper cross syndrome are other examples of postures that will stress the levator scapulae bilaterally. It is important, however, to consider the unilateral influences of this muscle where one side is lengthened and the other is shortened as well.

Posterior Muscles of the Upper Back and Thorax

The serratus posterior superior and the serratus posterior inferior fit best in this chapter because they attach to the ribs and play a role in breathing by controlling movement of the ribs in inhalation and exhalation, respectively. Both muscles are highly proprioceptive (figure 7.1). When the scapula is malpositioned, it can compress the serratus posterior superior, leading to pain under the scapula.

Serratus Posterior Superior

Origin
Spinous processes of C7 through T2 or T3
Ligamentum nuchae

Insertion
Superior borders of ribs 2 through 5, lateral to the angle

Action
Elevation of the upper ribs

Innervation
Anterior primary rami of nerves T1 through T4

Stressor Considerations

The serratus posterior superior functions as part of deep inhalation to open the ribs, creating more space in the thoracic cavity. The muscle fibers are highly proprioceptive and sensitive to changes in the thoracic cavity, firing to prevent excessive movement of the ribs; they thereby control pressure changes in the cavity and, in turn, the amount of air allowed into the lungs. The proprioception serves as a secondary check of the breathing mechanism. Stressors for the serratus posterior superior include situations in which (a) excessive deep inhalations are taken and (b) the muscle is recruited as part of breathing dysfunctions when the normally recruited breathing muscles are not functioning correctly. Given that the serratus posterior superior is more proprioceptive than strong, it is prone to myofascial dysfunction when overused.

Based on its location, the serratus posterior superior is subject to compression when scapular dysfunction occurs. The serratus posterior superior attaches directly on the ribs where it is deep to both the trapezius and rhomboids and slides underneath the scapulae. As mentioned throughout chapters 4 and 6, mispositioning of the scapulae in protraction can cause numerous issues. With the serratus posterior superior, protraction of the scapulae can result in compression, which leads to trigger points and myofascial dysfunction. Pain underneath the scapulae associated with painful breathing is a sign of compression of the serratus posterior superior and the associated dysfunction. Again, manual therapy treatment

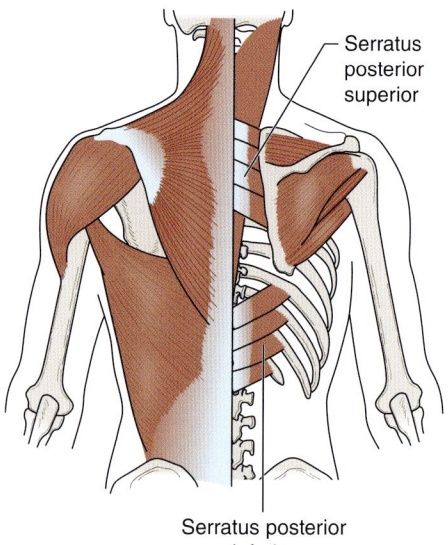

Figure 7.1 The serratus posterior superior is visible angling inferiorly on the ribs as it slides under the scapula while the serratus posterior superior angles superiorly from the vertebrae to the ribs.

to relieve this pain involves releasing the scapular protractors and working through the trapezius and rhomboids, as well as attempting to work underneath the medial border of the scapula to indirectly reduce myofascial pain.

Serratus Posterior Inferior

Origin
Spinous processes of T10 through L3

Insertion
Inferior border of ribs 9 through 12, lateral to the angle

Action
Draws the last four ribs downward and outward, countering the pull of the diaphragm

Innervation
Branches from the anterior primary rami of T9 through T12

Stressor Considerations

The serratus posterior inferior is used in deep exhalation to counter the pull of the diaphragm, preventing the ribs from being pulled upward. Like its cousin, the serratus posterior superior, the serratus posterior inferior is a flat muscle that is highly proprioceptive and not very strong. Because exhalation is passive, the serratus posterior inferior is not engaged frequently in normal, quiet breathing and is not typically affected if the breathing dysfunction involves inhalation only. Stressors include situations in which deep exhalations occur frequently or when the diaphragm cannot be engaged to its full capacity. If there is myofascial dysfunction in the area, the serratus posterior inferior may be compromised secondarily, such as with dysfunction in the latissimus dorsi, to which the serratus posterior inferior is deep. Low back pain associated with painful breathing may indicate a need to treat the serratus posterior inferior, even if breathing dysfunction is not noted.

Posterior Cervical Muscles

The muscles in the posterior cervical region, which include the trapezius and the levator scapulae, are involved in extension, lateral flexion, and rotation of the neck (figure 7.2). In addition, we have the splenius cervicis and splenius capitis muscles that laterally flex and rotate the neck to the same side and the semispinalis cervicis and capitis that extend the head and neck and perform rotation of the neck to the opposite side. Although people think of the neck as one structure, the neck has right and left sides, with sets of muscles on either side working bilaterally (e.g., with neck extension) and unilaterally (e.g., with lateral flexion and rotation). Therefore, it is not unusual for each side of the neck to respond differently to stressors. For example, a right-handed baseball pitcher who tends to whip his head around when he throws may have pain on the left side of his neck that is unrelated to his throwing mechanics at the shoulder but would still cause problems.

Splenius Cervicis and Capitis

Origin

Splenius cervicis: spinous processes of T3 through T6

Splenius capitis: lower half of the nuchal ligaments and spinous processes of C7 through T2

Insertion

Splenius cervicis: transverse processes of C1 through C3

Splenius capitis: mastoid process of the skull and lateral third of the superior nuchal line

Action

Bilaterally provide extension of the head (splenius capitis) and neck (splenius cervicis)

Unilaterally provide lateral flexion and ipsilateral rotation of the cervical spine

Innervation

Posterior rami of the spinal nerves

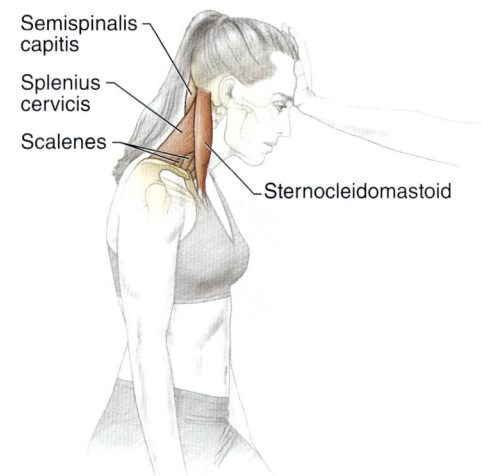

Figure 7.2 A lateral view of the semispinalis capitis and the splenius cervicis as they wrap around the neck along with views of the anterior muscles, the scalenes, and the sternocleidomastoid.

Stressor Considerations

The splenius muscles sit deep to the trapezius in the cervical region. Like many of the spinal muscles, they control both the head and neck and are difficult to differentiate on palpation, although differentiation is not necessary because they are treated together. Spanning between the spinous processes and transverse processes, the splenii hang out in the lamina groove. The splenii are extensors of the head and neck, and stressors include forward head posture and hyperextension of the head. Considerations should be made to treat both the neck and head if the splenii muscles are suspected to be involved in the problem. Positions in which the head is consistently rotated to the same side will also lead to dysfunction, with the affected side shortened and the contralateral side lengthened. Examples of stressors leading to rotation of the head can include sleeping positions (e.g., stomach sleeping and turning the head to one side) and computer monitor positioning to the side, forcing a head turn. With rotational considerations, it is important to treat the right and left sides as antagonists to each other.

Semispinalis Cervicis and Capitis

Origin

Semispinalis cervicis: transverse processes T1 through T5 or T6

Semispinalis capitis: transverse processes C4 through T7

Insertion

Semispinalis cervicis: spinous processes C2 through C5

Semispinalis capitis: occipital bone between the superior and inferior nuchal lines

Action

Extension and contralateral rotation of the vertebrae (semispinalis cervicis) and the head (semispinalis capitis)

Innervation

Posterior primary ramus of the same-level spinal nerve

Stressor Considerations

The semispinalis is part of the transversospinalis group (see chapter 8) that has a large presence in the cervical and capitis regions. Therefore, the semispinalis makes another appearance in this chapter. It is often implicated in pain and dysfunction in the head and neck. Stressors of the other posterior cervical muscles apply to the semispinalis as well.

Upper Back Treatment

There is some crossover in treating the upper back using treatments for the shoulder (chapter 6) and low back (chapter 8), because the muscles are continuous in these three areas. Because of the crossover between the upper back and the low back and shoulders, if you are not having success with what you are using from here, be sure to check one of the other chapters for additional ideas.

Warming of the upper back can be done with compressions and some fascial spreading (using the hands in opposite directions along the back to elicit a stretch). While facing into the table, place your hands on the client's back, using the heel of your hand or a loose fist to engage the tissue. For compressions, you can engage and twist your hand or fist. For fascial spreading, lay your entire hand on the client's back with each hand crossed, facing the opposite direction. As you engage in the tissue, create a pull in opposing directions with your hands as the fascia guides them apart (do not force this; let the fascia pull your hands). This general warm-up need not focus on any specific structure; rather, it provides an opportunity to increase blood flow to warm the tissues. The warm-up can be done to the entire back region before moving to specific treatments of the upper back musculature. The time spent warming and engaging the tissues can also be used for palpation purposes to note any areas of tension or restriction that may not have been obvious from the initial clinician intake and history.

Specific treatment for the upper back starts with the trapezius as the most superficial muscle. Glides along the trapezius are initiated in relation to the fiber direction of the muscle (figure 7.3). To release the upper trapezius, start with glides on the lower trapezius. Using a palm or loose fist, work between the medial border of the scapula and the spinous processes, starting at the level of the spine of the scapula down to the 12th vertebra and rib. Glides should have slow engagement into the fascia. For movement, add passive abduction of the humerus, lifting the arm up while gliding down the lower trapezius. This technique will make it easier to address the upper trapezius both at the superior aspect of the shoulder and the posterior aspect of the neck. For the upper portion of the trapezius along the top of the shoulder, the muscle curls around as it attaches between the spinous processes and the lateral third of the clavicle. If the muscle is warm enough, you can use one hand and work to unroll the trapezius by grasping the portion that curls over the top of the shoulder while engaging the lower portions of the muscle (figure 7.4). This technique works to relieve tension from holding the shoulders up (elevation of the scapula). Remembering to work the lower trapezius first will make it easier to engage the postural upper portion.

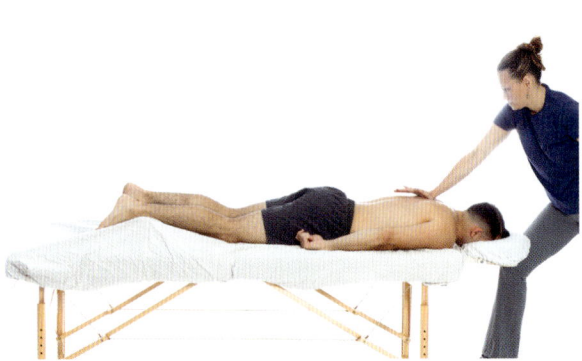

Figure 7.3 The heel of the hand is used along the trapezius to provide myofascial glides. The intent of the movement is caudally (toward the tailbone) to help counter the eccentric strain of the lower trapezius muscles.

As a scapular retractor, the middle trapezius runs more linear from the spinous processes to the acromion process of the scapula. The fibers will likely be influenced by the manual therapy treatments for the upper and lower trapezius; however, it does not hurt to do a few glides in the area before working the deeper muscles. Once the trapezius has been treated, it becomes warm enough to allow work through the rhomboids, which angle from the spinous processes to the medial border of the scapula. Changing the approach to the glides from more linear to an angle will address the rhomboids instead of the middle trapezius. As mentioned previously, the rhomboids are phasic, meaning they are eccentrically lengthened and do not need to be stretched. However, by adding passive movement to the glides, the eccentrically contracted muscle fibers can be encouraged to release with the fascia. This release is achieved with passive shortening of the rhomboids by lifting the arm into horizontal abduction, thereby retracting the scapula, then gliding from the medial border of the scapula toward the spinous processes on an angle distally to proximally while slowly bringing the arm down (figure 7.5). As the rhomboids attach to the medial border of the scapula, work across the table to access the medial border and add some cross-fiber friction over the attachments. By working this area, it becomes easier to lift and mobilize the scapula.

Lifting and mobilizing the scapula can help to reach the next layer, the serratus posterior superior. Serratus posterior superior muscle fibers have the same fiber direction as the rhomboid major, just one layer deeper, and the muscle fibers run under the scapula. If the scapula can be mobilized enough to provide some glides underneath the medial border, through the rhomboid and the trapezius muscles , then

Chapter 7 Upper Back and Neck

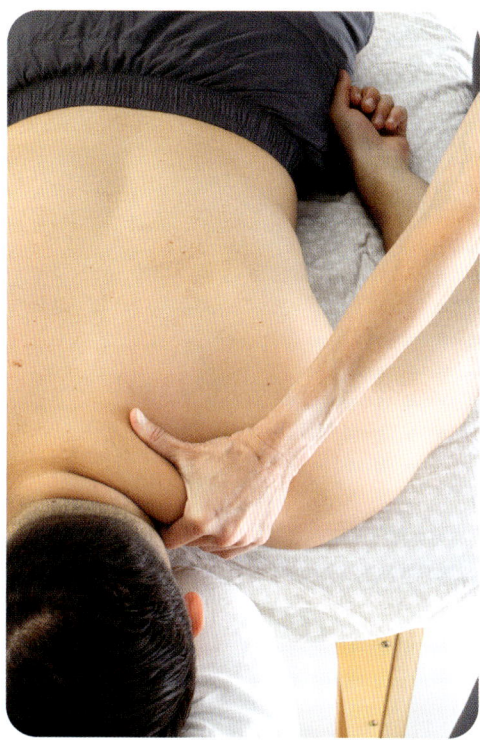

Figure 7.4 Unrolling the trapezius. The fingers of one hand are curled around the muscle, lifting it up and off the clavicle while drawing it toward the tailbone (caudally).

some additional work to the serratus posterior superior can be provided. This treatment may not be warranted for all patients, however; for patients experiencing any of the stressors listed earlier for the serratus posterior superior, this treatment is a great way to relieve discomfort.

Not listed here are treatments for the erector spinae group in the thoracic region, which are outlined in chapter 8 as part of the start of the back treatment. Addressing these muscles may be important for treating the thoracic spine and for relieving the cervical spine if the issue is related to the erectors. Instead of repeating the information here, visit chapter 8 for more details on the treatment.

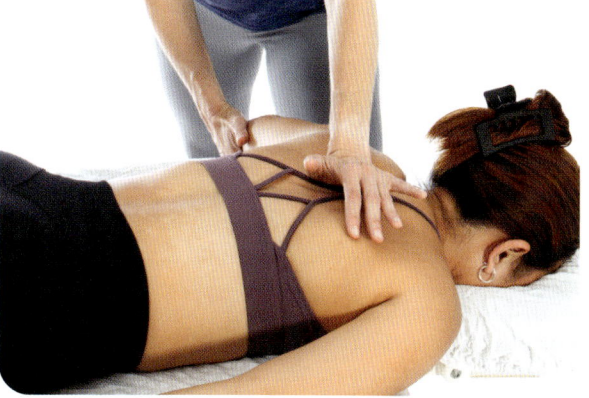

Figure 7.5 The rhomboids are passively shortened with the arm in horizontal abduction and scapular retraction; the arm is slowly lowered as the therapist performs glides toward the vertebrae.

Prone Neck Treatment

The part of the upper trapezius that resides in the neck, as well as the rest of the cervical extensors, can be treated with the patient in a prone, supine, or seated position. It is not necessary to do all the treatments in each position every session. It is preferrable to do what works best in the situation, what adequately addresses the patient's goals and a bit of clinical reasoning. For example, if the clinician is providing treatment to the back, the prone treatment might be preferred over the supine treatment. If the client is having trouble lying face down, the supine position might be preferred. The prone treatment can be done after the upper back treatment or before or even in the middle of it; just make sure to warm the areas before beginning the more specific treatment.

The patient should be positioned prone with the neck straight, preferably supported in a face cradle or a prone pillow on the table. It is important for the patient's head and neck to be supported for this work; if this is not possible, consider one of the seated or supine techniques. Position yourself at the top of the table in a stable lunge position with one foot in front of the other. You can lean a little more to one side of the head or the other as needed. Warm the superficial fascia with some gentle compressive finger circles on either side of the spinous processes in the lamina groove. Because of the patient's head position, ensure you do not push down into the neck; rather, engage the fascia along the muscle linearly. Your circles should extend through the lamina groove between the prominent T1 spinous process and the external occipital protuberance, working up and down the length of the neck.

Lifting and shifting of the fascia can be used to release the ligamentum nuchae, a fascial attachment for the muscles in the cervical spine (figure 7.6). Picking up the fascia (e.g., think of grabbing a cat by the scruff of the neck) is done by placing both of your hands together, then lifting the fascia and shifting superiorly and inferiorly as well as medially and laterally. Sometimes the patient will try to help by bringing their neck into flexion, which makes it harder for you to perform the treatment. Communication is key to having the patient positioned correctly. In addition, communicate clearly about pressure, because the techniques should not be performed with a lot of downward pressure.

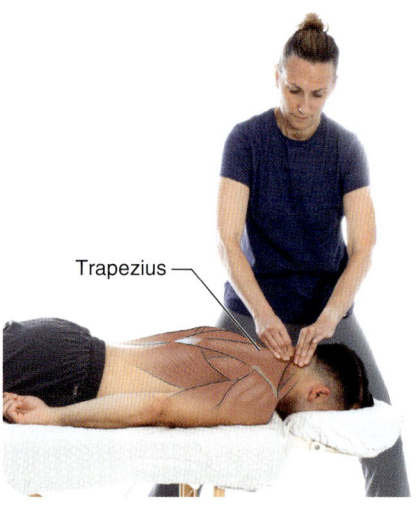

Figure 7.6 Lifting and shifting of the fascia of the posterior neck with the patient in a prone position.

Suboccipital Muscles

Four suboccipital muscles serve to control the head on the neck: the rectus capitis posterior major, the rectus capitis posterior minor, the obliquus capitis superior, and the obliquus capitis inferior (figure 7.7). These muscles are specifically responsible for movements between the occiput and C1 (atlantooccipital joint) and between C1 and C2 (atlantoaxial joint). Essentially, they provide the movements of extension, lateral flexion, and rotation of the head on the neck.

Rectus Capitis Posterior Major

Origin
 Spinous process of C2 (axis)

Insertion
 Lateral portion of the inferior nuchal line of the occipital bone

Action
 Extension of the head (atlantooccipital joint)
 Rotation of the head to the same side (atlantoaxial joint)

Innervation
 Posterior rami of C1

Rectus Capitis Posterior Minor

Origin
 Posterior tubercle of C1

Insertion
 Medial portion of the inferior nuchal line of the occipital bone

Action
 Extension of the head (atlantooccipital joint)

Innervation
 Posterior rami of C1

Obliquus Capitis Superior

Origin
 Transverse process of C1

Insertion
 Occipital bone between the inferior and superior nuchal lines

Action
  Extension and lateral flexion of the head (atlantooccipital joint)

Innervation
  Posterior rami of C1

Obliquus Capitis Inferior

Origin
  Spinous process of C2

Insertion
  Transverse process of the atlas

Action
  Rotation of the atlantoaxial joint

Innervation
  Posterior rami of C1

Stressor Considerations

The suboccipital muscles are very small and involved in finite movement of the head on the neck. Stressors for these muscles rarely come from overuse; rather, they come from compression of or hyperextension of the head on neck. Based on the *righting reflex*, these muscles are compressed with forward head posture, such as when someone hyperextends the head to look at the horizon. Complicating the compression of these muscles is the vertebral artery running through the suboccipital triangle. The *suboccipital triangle* is made up of the rectus capitis posterior major, the obliquus capitis inferior, and the obliquus capitis superior. The vertebral artery runs through the transverse foramen in the transverse processes of the cervical vertebrae, sits on top of C1, and then runs through the suboccipital triangle to join the posterior aspect of the circle of Willis, the ring of arteries located at the base of the brain. When the muscles (which are postural) respond to stress, they shorten and widen, closing the space within the triangle. Decreasing the space where the blood vessel travels can put pressure on the vessel, which, in turn, can lead to headaches. Treatment of these muscles can help open the space and relieve muscle tension contributing to headaches.

The four suboccipitals are another example of muscles that are not very strong but are very specialized and highly proprioceptive as they work to keep the eyes level and the head positioned optimally. An additional stressor of these muscles with sport is any situation that can upset this proprioceptive response. For example, the mechanism that leads to concussion can jar these muscles, causing dysfunction; the resulting dysfunction of the cranial nerves following a concussion can result in compensatory responses that will stress these muscles. (It is important to note that although this muscle dysfunction is a result of what occurs with a concussion, in no way is any of this discussion intended to substitute for appropriate care of the neurological components of a head injury.) Treatment in this area may assist with decreasing postconcussion symptoms by allowing the head to make its fine-tuned adjustments.

Chapter 7 Upper Back and Neck

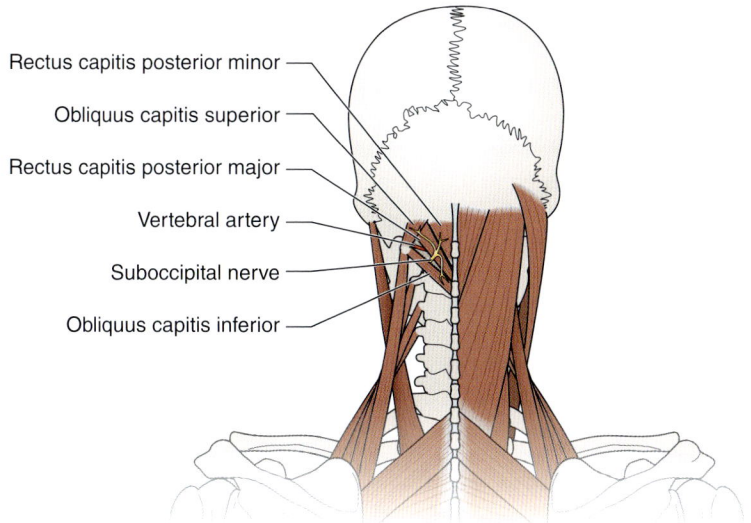

Figure 7.7 The four suboccipital muscles span the space between the occipital bone of the skull, C1, and C2. The vertebral artery goes through the *suboccipital triangle,* made up of the rectus capitis posterior major, the obliquus capitis inferior, and the obliquus capitis superior, on its way to the brain.

Anterior Cervical Muscles

The muscles of the anterior neck act in flexion of the cervical spine as well as in rotation and lateral flexion (figure 7.8). The anterior cervical muscles also play a role in breathing, with attachments to the ribs and sternum. Although patients rarely complain of anterior neck pain, treatment in this area will help balance the posterior neck and upper back pain. Because of the presence of arteries, nerves, and the trachea, caution must be used when treating this area.

Sternocleidomastoid

Origin
  Manubrium of the sternum
  Medial one-third of the clavicle

Insertion
  Mastoid process of the skull

Action
  Bilaterally produces flexion of the cervical spine
  Unilaterally produces lateral flexion and contralateral rotation of the cervical spine

Innervation
  Accessory nerve (cranial nerve XI)

Stressor Considerations

The sternocleidomastoid has stressors related to all its attachments. Attaching on the sternum means the sternocleidomastoid can be negatively affected by compensatory breathing patterns. The sternocleidomastoid's insertion on the mastoid process is a biomechanically stressed area because it shares this attachment with the longissimus (of the erector spinae group) and the splenius capitis, all of which pull in different directions. In addition, the muscle belly sits on the carotid artery, meaning caution must be taken to not compress the artery during treatment (lifting of the fascia is better than compressive techniques for this muscle). The muscle may also be stressed with jarring-type mechanisms, such as events that can lead to concussion. Also, trigger points in the sternocleidomastoid can lead to dizziness and nausea, making it important for clinicians to communicate with the patient so as not to end a treatment if these symptoms begin on the table (Travell and Simons 1983). These stressors occur aside from its action, flexion of the neck, where the sternocleidomastoid becomes shortened as part of forward head posture, and its actions of contralateral rotation and lateral flexion, which share stressors as described in the section on the posterior neck muscles.

Scalenes

Origin
Anterior: transverse processes of C3 through C6
Middle: transverse processes of C2 through C7
Posterior: transverse processes of C5 through C7

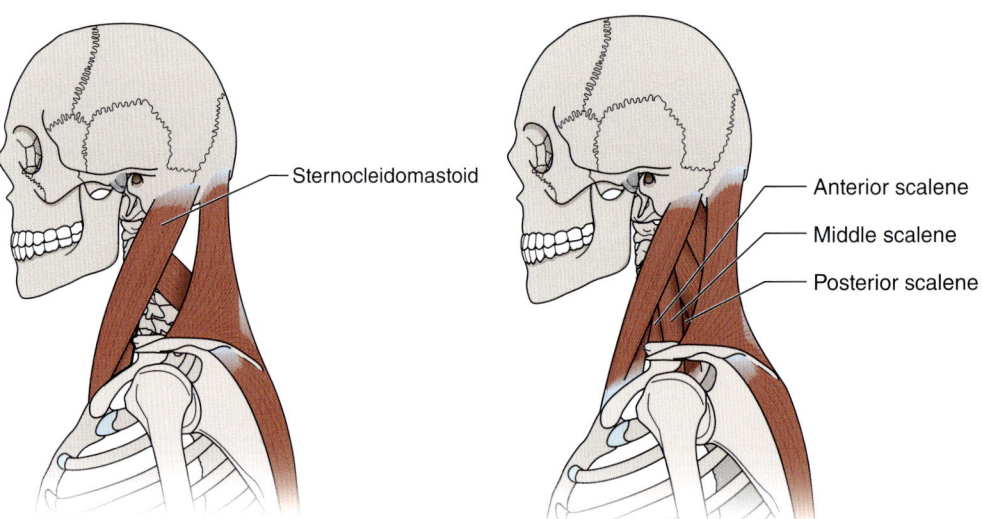

Figure 7.8 Both images show lateral views of the neck muscles. *(a)* The sternocleidomastoid can be seen running from the manubrium of the sternum and the clavicle to the mastoid process on the skull. *(b)* The scalene muscles sit lateral and deep to the sternocleidomastoid, running from the transverse processes of the cervical vertebrae to the ribs.

Insertion
   Anterior: inner border and upper surface of rib 1
   Middle: superior surface of rib 1
   Posterior: outer surface of rib 2

Action
   Flexion, lateral flexion, and contralateral rotation of the cervical spine
   Anterior and middle scalenes elevate rib 1
   Posterior scalene elevates rib 2

Innervation
   Ventral rami of C5 and C6 (anterior), C3 through C8 (middle), and C6 through C8 (posterior)

Stressor Considerations

The scalene muscles are associated with forward head posture stressors as well as breathing-related stressors. As a flexor of the neck, the scalene muscles are shortened bilaterally with forward head posture. Unilaterally, the scalene muscles can be shortened with lateral flexion on one side and lengthened or eccentrically strained on the other. With contralateral rotation, the muscles become shortened on the opposite side to which they are rotated (and lengthened on the same side). These considerations again reinforce the need for clinicians to work bilaterally, especially if they forget which muscles are contralateral rotators and which are ipsilateral rotators.

The scalene muscles serve as accessory breathing muscles in inhalation, pulling the ribs superiorly to help expand the space in the thoracic cavity. With improper breathing in which the diaphragm is not used properly by flattening, (thereby increasing space and decreasing pressure in the thoracic cavity), the scalene muscles will take up the slack, pulling upward to create more space. This dysfunctional breathing pattern leads to myofascial dysfunction. If this pattern is combined with forward head posture, both the scalene muscles and the ability to take deep breaths become deficient. Performing artists, such as singers and musicians who play a wind instrument, may have overdeveloped scalene muscles, secondary to their breathing habits. If the instrument requires positioning the head and neck in a way that stresses the scalene muscles and the sternocleidomastoid, considerations should be taken to treat the muscles to relieve the resulting myofascial dysfunction.

Supine Neck Treatment

The supine position has advantages for working the posterior aspect of the neck, because the neck can be supported on the table. Although this position alleviates concerns such as pushing down into the unsupported neck, it does not give clinicians a license to use too much pressure on the structures. Another advantage is the clinician can use the weight of the head and neck to create the pressure, as opposed to using the fingers or thumbs to push into the structures. To start, position the patient supine on the table with their head and neck lying on (supported by) the table. Sit at the head of the table, either on a chair or stool, with your feet firmly planted on the floor. In the absence of a stool or chair, you can use a kneeling position. In the kneeling position, place your hands under the patient's head and neck on the table so they are resting on your hands. This position alleviates the need to support the head, meaning you do not have to work as hard.

You can once again use prone gentle circles in the lamina groove between T1 and the external occipital protuberance to warm the area. Glides can be done in the lamina groove using your thumb, one side at a time (figure 7.9). Hold the client's head in the opposite hand of the one you will be using for glides (you will be using the hand on the same side as which you are working). To start, turn the client's head away from the side you are working. Gently glide your thumb along the lamina groove, using the opposite hand to turn the client's head into the thumb and thereby controlling the pressure. Remember, during all of this, both of your hands are on the table and the client's head is in your hands. Avoid doing more work yourself by holding the head up. If the client tries to hold their head up, nicely remind them not to work so hard because they are engaging the muscles you are trying to release.

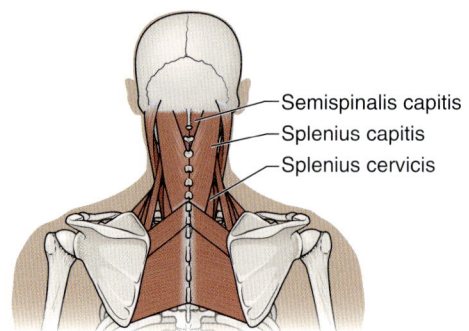

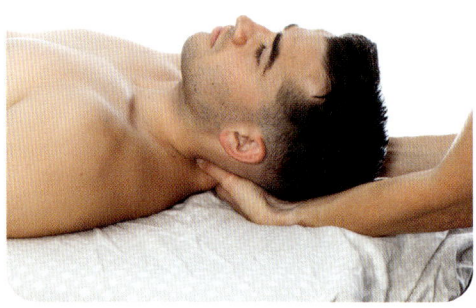

Figure 7.9 The therapist uses the side of the thumb to glide in the lamina groove, between the spinous processes and the transverse processes.

To work the suboccipital muscles, use the same position just described, with the patient supine on the table and their head resting on your hands Sit at the head of the table. Take your hands around the head, using your fingers, and find the patient's superior nuchal line, which juts out on either side of the external occipital protuberance. Start with gentle circles to warm the area before proceeding. For the technique, slide the fingers along the occipital bone, following the curve of the skull until you reach the space between the nuchal lines (you can feel the fingertips sink into the muscle and fascia). With the patient's head in your hands and your hands on the table, let the weight of the head provide the pressure as your fingers sink up into the suboccipital muscles (figure 7.10a). To increase the pressure, gently turn the patient's head into one hand (figure 7.10b). Let your fingertips sink into the area to release. Repeat on the other side.

Work with the anterior neck should be done with care (see the Anterior Neck Cautions sidebar). Positioning is the same, with the patient supine and you seated at the head of the table. The patient's head should be laterally flexed and rotated to the side being worked to give the muscles some slack away from the neurovascular structures.

For the sternocleidomastoid, avoid direct pressure to the muscle belly. Attend to the attachments as well as the fascia covering the muscle. To begin treating the sternocleidomastoid, use gentle finger circles or glides just at the mastoid process

Chapter 7 Upper Back and Neck

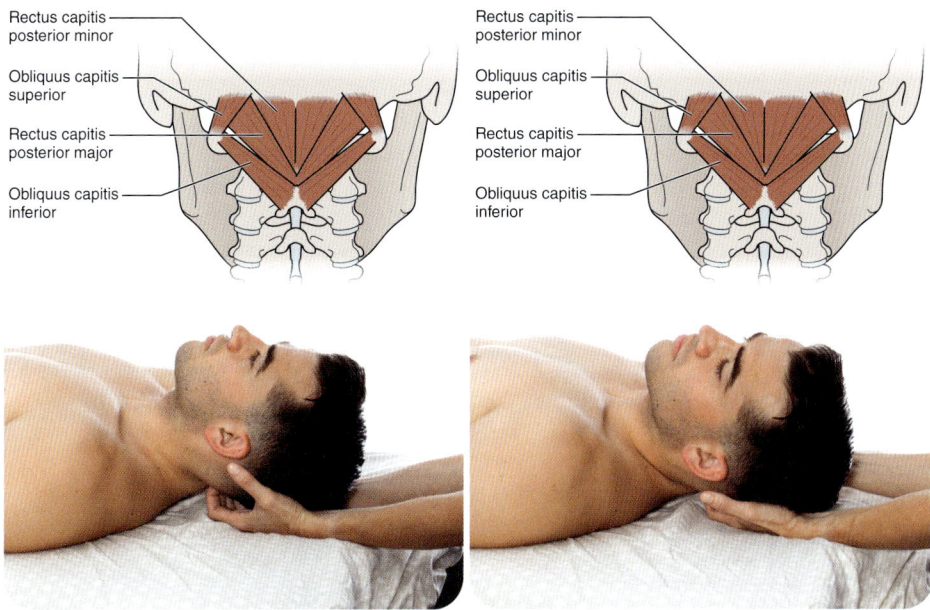

Figure 7.10 *(a)* The fingertips are placed gently in the suboccipital space with the clinician's arms on the table and the head supported. *(b)* The head is rotated to the side to provide more pressure, coming from the weight of the skull and not any increased pressure by the therapist.

of the temporal bone to relieve stress at the area. To find the mastoid process, go to the most posterior part of the ear and slide straight down to the tender bone. Be sure to avoid moving too far anterior from the mastoid process, because the styloid process sits directly behind the earlobe. The styloid process of the temporal bone is very sensitive and is considered an endangerment site. Gentle circles, along with very short glides, can be used to warm the area. At the origin of the two heads (the clavicle and the manubrium of the sternum), lift and shift the fascia right over the bone. The muscle is between the two points just worked. Treatment here can also include just lifting and shifting of the fascia over the muscle. Do not worry about treating the muscle belly so much as releasing the fascia. Repeat on the other side, remembering to turn the client's head to the side you are now working.

The scalene muscles sit just posterior to the sternocleidomastoid (in order: anterior, middle, and then posterior) with a slight space for the thoracic outlet between the middle and posterior scalenes. With the head positioned in slight lateral flexion and rotation, you can perform glides on the muscle, heading down to the first rib (anterior and middle scalenes) and the second rib (posterior scalene). Glide just along the muscle without pushing with deep pressure.

Cautions for the Anterior Neck

Because of the sensitive structures in the anterior neck, treatment needs to be precise over the affected muscles. Treatments must avoid putting pressure on the carotid artery and the trachea.

Seated Neck and Upper Back Treatment

The techniques described for the upper back and neck that are described in both the supine and prone positions can be performed with the patient in a seated position. The disadvantage is the patient holds up their head during the treatment, preventing complete relaxation of the muscles. A seated massage chair can be used but is not necessary. If you are using a massage chair, the patient may be forced into an exaggerated rounded shoulder position with the arms resting in front of the body. Position yourself standing behind the patient, using a lunge stance. You can use compressions to warm the upper back. You can use lifting and shifting of the posterior cervical muscles and unrolling of the upper trapezius to release the superficial layer.

As with the supine treatment, the weight of the client's head can be used to elicit pressure. Place one of your hands gently on the client's head, and place the thumb of your other hand in the lamina groove. Gently move the client's head onto your thumb to release the muscle in that area. Release the head and reposition the thumb around to reach a new space. Remember to release the head before moving the thumb to a new spot. The suboccipital muscles can also be worked with some gentle circles. Stand in front of the patient with the fingers in the suboccipital space, and use gentle traction of the head while sinking into the space. The key to the transfer of these techniques from the client in a prone or supine position to a seated position is to get creative with what you have while maintaining good body mechanics for yourself.

WHY DOES THE CLINICIAN CARE?

Upper back and neck pain is a common complaint for both athletes and nonathletes. People live in a world where they frequently use electronic devices (laptops, smartphones, tablets, and computers), making activities of daily living a potential cause of stress to the upper back and neck. Considering that many athletes are also students and many active individuals have day jobs, the positions individuals hold outside of sport can affect their ability to perform on the field. Think about typing on a laptop: How are the user's hands positioned? How does the user hold their head? Now think about engaging in a sport: What happens when someone picks up a ball to throw or a pickleball paddle? The body remembers these positions thanks to Davis' law. Relief to the eccentrically strained muscles of the upper back and the shortened cervical flexors is welcomed by all.

Lower Back and Abdomen

The lower back (lumbar) and abdominal regions provide support and power for the transfer of energy between the upper and lower body. Weakness and lack of endurance in this area can lead to injuries, both acute and overuse. In addition, weakness and lack of endurance above and below this area on the kinetic chain can cause the low back or abdomen to take on more stress. Lack of strength, endurance, and range of motion are often concerns. As discussed in this chapter, clinicians can create a manual therapy treatment to help balance the stress on the musculature.

Lumbar Spine Structure

The lumbar spine is composed of five large vertebrae resting on the top of the sacrum. The sacrum is made up of five fused bones and attaches to the coccyx, which is composed of two to five fused bones. The vertebrae in the lumbar region are very large and thick; they support the upper vertebrae and the weight of the head, and they also help absorb energy transferred from the lower extremity up the kinetic chain. Although the lumbar vertebrae allow for movement in all three planes, rotation is limited, with more motion occurring in the sagittal and frontal planes than in the transverse plane. As with the cervical and thoracic spine, range of motion comes from the aggregate movement of the vertebral segments on one another. If there are any limits in the available motion at a segment, the overall range of motion of the vertebral column can be compromised. Muscles in the lumbar region attach to the vertebrae as well as the iliac crest, sacrum, and lower ribs. The bony structure in this area is limited. The lack of bones to support the structures puts more stress on the soft tissue structures (muscles and fascia) to maintain integrity in this region.

Abdomen Structure

The abdomen has very little bony anatomy. Essentially, the abdomen comprises the anterior space between the lower ribs and the pubic bone. The abdominal muscles have bony attachments between the ribs, pubic bone, and iliac crest, with soft tissue attachments to the inguinal ligament, abdominal fascia, and thoracolumbar fascia. Because these muscles rely on fascia for their attachments and because fascia is reliant on the properties of tensegrity, stress to these muscles can result in pull in different directions. For example, a right-handed hitter in baseball will put stress on the right and left sides of the abdomen differently. The same can be seen for a golfer. Therefore, instead of working the body with antagonist muscles being anterior and posterior, clinicians would consider the muscles on the right and left sides as being antagonists.

Thoracolumbar Aponeurosis Structure

The *thoracolumbar aponeurosis* is a multilayered fascial structure separating the erector muscles, the quadratus lumborum, and the psoas major (figure 8.1). Depending on the source, the thoracolumbar aponeurosis can be considered to have two or three layers, serving as attachments for muscles from the lumbar, gluteal, and abdominal regions as well as the latissimus dorsi, a shoulder muscle (Willard et al. 2012). Because many of the muscles attaching here have opposing lines of pull, stress on the thoracolumbar aponeurosis can come from any of these areas. In addition, the stress from any of these areas will cause changes in an opposing area, owing to the properties of tensegrity in the fascia. For example, pull from the right latissimus dorsi will be opposed by the left gluteal region, making it important to apply manual therapy and train the muscles (e.g., with an opposite arm and leg movement) in both areas. As clinicians consider some of these postural alignment

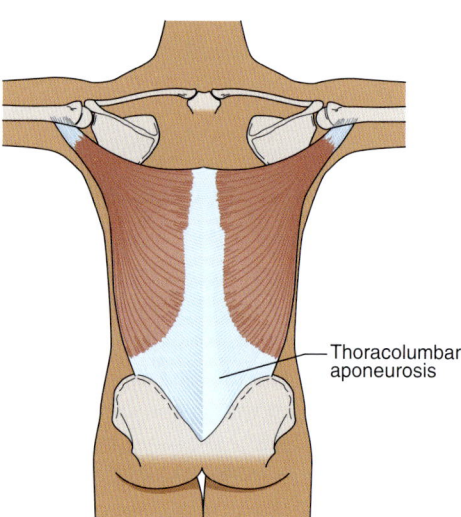

Figure 8.1 The thoracolumbar aponeurosis extends from the gluteal region through the lumbar and abdominal regions. This multi-layered structure serves as a site of muscle attachment as well as separating various layers of muscles in the region.

concerns, such as anterior or lateral pelvic tilt, the effects of these distortions on the thoracolumbar fascia need to be addressed.

Upper-Body and Lower-Body Considerations (Linking Above and Below)

When clinicians think about sports that are upper-extremity dominant, they must consider the transfer of energy from the lower body through the lower back and abdomen into the upper extremity. Picture a baseball pitcher stepping with his left foot to throw with his right arm, a volleyball player using a two-foot takeoff to hit or block, or a runner generating power from her legs and driving with her arms. Stability in the lower back and abdomen assists in keeping the pelvis stable, which is one of many ways to help prevent lower-extremity overuse injuries. These are just a few basic examples of the connection built from this region of the body and are considerations when providing treatment to these areas.

Right and Left Considerations (Linking Side to Side)

For the muscles of the axial skeleton, consideration must be given to the anterior and posterior muscles working as antagonists but also to the muscles on the right and left sides, as mentioned in this chapter and in the discussion of the neck in chapter 7. The right and left sides are called on to do different things, especially with rotational movements. Lateral flexion is a unilateral movement, but as one side flexes laterally, the other side will stretch. Rotational movements, which can even include bringing the arm across the body, cause one group of muscles to contract, while the other group will stretch. Consider this example with the abdominal obliques: The external obliques perform contralateral rotation while the internal obliques perform ipsilateral rotation. When someone turns to the left, the right external obliques and the left internal obliques produce a concentric contraction. During this motion, the left external obliques and the right internal obliques lengthen. Just as clinicians consider the anterior and posterior, they need to consider the right and left sides.

MUSCLES OF THE BACK AND ABDOMEN

The muscles in the lumbar region rely on very little bony anatomy to do their job; therefore, they are subject to the properties of tensegrity, relying on balance in each other to support the linking from the lower extremity to the upper extremity and vice versa. Considerations need to be made if the activity relies on transfer of energy up or down the kinetic chain (e.g., the difference between throwing a ball and swinging a bat). These muscles also have the unique trait of performing actions bilaterally (with the right and left sides contracting together) as well as unilaterally (with the right side or left side contracting). Bilateral activation of the muscles performs actions in the sagittal plane, whereas unilateral activation of the muscles performs actions in either the transverse or frontal plane. Movement of the joints results from aggregate movement of the spine. Therefore, some muscles, such those in the erector spinae group, cross multiple vertebral levels, a design intended to create movement of larger segments (e.g., three or more vertebrae). Other muscles, such as the rotatores of the deep transversospinalis group, focus on the smaller segment with the gliding movement of one or two vertebrae on each other.

Additionally, some of the muscles cross between the lumbar region into the thoracic and cervical region, making isolation (as well as remembering the full origin and insertion criteria) difficult. Therefore, treatment does not stop or start at L1. This chapter aims to discuss techniques typical to the entire back rather than separate regions.

Posterior Lumbar Region

The posterior lumbar region is covered by the thoracolumbar fascia and the latissimus dorsi, an extrinsic shoulder muscle. Therefore, treatment must start with warming through these superficial structures. The posterior muscles consist of the erector spinae, the superficial erector spinae group controlling the movements at the vertebrae, and the deep transversospinalis group, controlling rotation of the vertebrae at various segment levels. The main muscle of concern with low back pain, however, is the quadratus lumborum. Depending on the activity, the quadratus lumborum can either move the lumbar spine on the more stable pelvis or move the pelvis on the more stable lumbar spine.

Erector Spinae Group

The erector spinae group is located between the spinous and transverse processes in the lamina groove, deep within the thoracolumbar fascia (figure 8.2). From medial to lateral, it includes the spinalis, the longissimus, and the iliocostalis. The spinalis is located in the thoracic and cervical region only, whereas the longissimus is found in the thoracic and cervical regions and extends to the head (capitis). Therefore, only the iliocostalis is found in the lumbar region. However, the erector spinae group is covered here because the treatment is continuous along the length of the vertebral column.

Origin
　Sacrum
　Iliac crest
　Lower thoracic and lumbar spinous processes

Insertion
　Ribs and spinous processes of the upper thoracic and cervical vertebrae
　Longissimus inserts as high as the mastoid process of the skull

Action
　Bilaterally produces extension of the spine
　Unilaterally produces lateral flexion; functions in eccentric control of trunk flexion

Innervation
　Posterior branch of the spinal nerve at the associated level

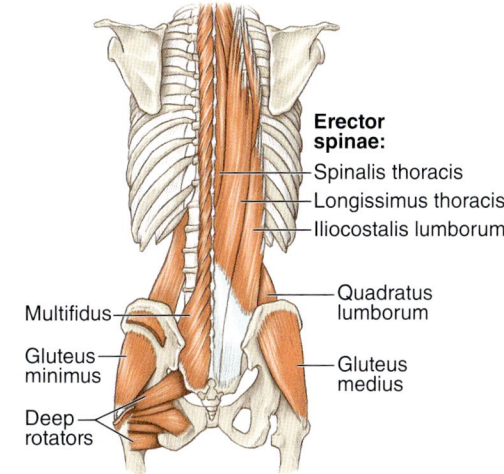

Figure 8.2 The erector spinae group (right); the multifidus, a deep rotator (left); the quadratus lumborum (bilateral); and the gluteal muscles. All of these muscles should be considered in the treatment of low back pain.

Stressor Considerations

The erector spinae group, while producing extension of the spine, functions to keep the body upright against gravity, controlling eccentric flexion of the spine. During movement, the erector spinae help to stabilize the spine, preventing excessive motion, which would not only have a detrimental effect on technique in sport but would also expend energy and thus contribute to early systemic fatigue. The erector spinae help distribute the load among the vertebral column, reducing stress on individual vertebrae and intervertebral discs and thereby decreasing injury risk. The erector spinae are predominantly slow twitch, highly anaerobic, and slow to fatigue, meaning these muscles can work for long periods to maintain stability when they are functioning properly. However, if other muscles are not functioning correctly, including the multifidus and the abdominals, the erector spinae group may be forced to take on extra load, thereby increasing the risk of fatigue, injury to the area, or mechanical breakdown. Understanding the role of the erector spinae and how to help these muscles maintain correct positioning is integral in not only addressing back pain but also maintaining proper function of the rest of the body.

Transversospinalis Muscle Group

The transversospinalis muscle group is deep to the erector spinae group (figure 8.2). They are sometimes referred to as the *gutter muscles*, sitting between the transverse processes and spinous processes, almost directly on the bone. As opposed to the erector spinae group that sits medially to laterally on the same layer, the transversospinalis muscles are layered from superficial to deep in the following order: the semispinalis, the multifidus, and the rotatores. The three layers also differ in the number of vertebrae they span. The semispinalis spans four to six vertebrae, the multifidus spans two to four vertebrae, and the rotatores span one to two vertebrae. The multifidus has a large presence in the lumbar region, and it is the only muscle of this group to be called out for a treatment in this chapter; therefore, it is given its own subsection here as well.

Semispinalis and Rotatores

Origin
　Transverse process of each vertebra

Insertion
　Rotatores: spinous processes of the vertebrae one to two levels above
　Semispinalis: spinous processes of the vertebrae four to six levels above

Action
　Bilaterally produces extension of the vertebral column
　Unilaterally produces contralateral rotation of the vertebral column

Innervation
　Posterior primary ramus of the spinal nerve at that level

Multifidus

Origin
　Sacrum
　Iliac spine
　Transverse processes of the vertebrae

Insertion
　Spinous processes of the vertebrae two to four levels above

Action
　Bilaterally produces extension of the vertebral column
　Unilaterally produces contralateral rotation of the vertebral column

Innervation
　Posterior primary ramus of the spinal nerve at that level

Stressor Considerations

Compared with the rest of the muscles in the lumbar region, the multifidus has the potential to be highly developed. When activated correctly, the multifidus serves to control the individual vertebrae maintaining proper alignment, to support the spine in upright posture, and to assist in controlling movements by the synergists and antagonists in the area. These benefits serve to decrease low back pain. When the multifidus is weak, fails to fire, or is altered in composition (as can happen with age), there is an increased risk of low back pain. Although strengthening is important, relieving myofascial dysfunction can also help alleviate symptoms. Reducing myofascial restrictions or trigger points can allow the muscle to work efficiently and potentially reduce pain, which will also improve function. Correct and efficient function of the multifidus, along with strengthening of the low back, can create more efficient stability in the vertebral column.

The semispinalis and the rotatores are stressed with movement at the individual vertebrae level. These muscles contribute to spinal stability more than producing great movements; therefore, they can be compromised, such as with facet joint syndrome. In addition, weakness or atrophy of these muscles can lead to compromised movement of the individual vertebral segment.

Quadratus Lumborum

Origin
Posterior anterior aspect of the iliac crest

Transverse processes of the lumbar vertebrae

Insertion
Inferior border of the 12th rib

Transverse processes of the lumbar vertebrae

Action
Bilaterally acts to expand the lumbar spine and stabilize the pelvis
Unilaterally acts to laterally flex the lumbar spine when the hip is stable and to elevate the hip when the torso is stable

Innervation
Branches of the T12 and L1 nerves

Stressor Considerations

The quadratus lumborum has fibers running from the iliac crest to the lumbar transverse processes, from the iliac crest to the 12th rib, and from the lumbar transverse processes to the 12th rib. This multilayered arrangement allows for stability and movement between the 12th rib, iliac crest, and lumbar vertebrae. Spasm or tension in the quadratus lumborum can lead to low back pain, rotation of the pelvis, and even pain with breathing, because the muscle attaches to the 12th rib. For these and many more reasons, the quadratus lumborum is often the source of low back pain. Unilateral shortening of the quadratus lumborum leads to a lateral pelvic tilt, whereas bilateral shortening leads to an anterior pelvic tilt. Habits such as using the hip to carry an object or a child can lead to a lateral pelvic tilt. Foot and gait adjustments, such as those made for hyperpronation or a leg-length discrepancy, can lead to unilateral shortening of the quadratus lumborum on the short side and lengthening on the long side. Seated postures that force one hip higher than the other can also be implicated. Although muscular low back pain can have a variety of causes, learning to treat the quadratus lumborum and the multifidus with manual therapy, stretching, and rehabilitation can help mitigate most muscular low back pain symptoms.

Low Back Prone Treatment

You can warm the lower back with compressions and fascial spreading. Face into the table and place your hands on the client's back, using the heel of the hand or your loose fist. For compressions, you can engage and twist your hand or fist. For fascial spreading to elicit a stretch, lay both of your hands on the client's back; the hands should be crossed, facing the opposite direction. As you engage in the tissue, create a pull in opposing directions with your hands as the fascia guides your hands apart (do not force this; let the fascia pull your hands). This general warm-up need not focus on any specific structure; it helps increase blood flow to warm the tissues. Additionally, you can use the warming noted with the abdominal treatment in the Abdominal Spiraling sidebar.

Although this section is specific to the low back, recall the anatomy of the erector spinae group mentioned earlier as well as the latissimus dorsi (chapter 6) and the trapezius (chapters 6 and 7) described previously. You can perform the warm-up for the entire back region before moving to specific treatments of the low back musculature. The time spent warming and engaging the tissues can also be used for palpation purposes, to note any areas of tension or restriction that may not have been obvious from the initial clinician intake and history.

The erector spinae group can be treated with myofascial glides in the lamina groove (figure 8.3). When you are standing on the same side of the table, a loose fist or the heel of your hand from the arm closest to the table works best. For the low back, you can begin the glides at the sacrum and work up the length of the spine. If your focus is more on the upper back or thoracic region, you can use the same technique to glide from the shoulder down the table while standing at the head of the table. Regardless of which direction you

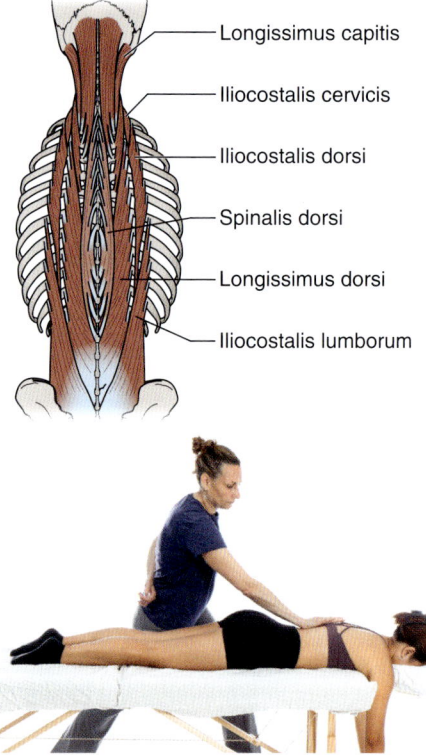

Figure 8.3 Glides are performed on the erector spinae muscles as part of the back treatment.

are working, engage with the fascia (not using lubricant) and let the fascia pull the hand (or fist) away from you. Either lunge forward with your legs as your arm slides, or step forward as you work the full range of the erectors. As a variation, you can face the table to work the erectors on the side opposite of where you are standing. Use the heel of your hand to traction the muscles off the spinous processes, reducing myofascial restrictions in the lamina groove. This technique can be done the length of the erectors, from sacrum to the shoulders, and on both the right and left sides. Remember to move your feet up or down the table as you work the corresponding portion of the erectors. Avoid reaching if you cannot balance yourself with your hips driving your arms.

Treatment for the multifidus, which is prominent in the low back, can be done after warming and glides. Standing at the level of the patient's iliac crest, position yourself facing toward the patient's head in a lunge position (figure 8.4). Find the patient's posterior superior iliac spine (PSIS), the top of the sacrum, and the lower two spinous processes (L4 and L5). Line up the olecranon of your inside arm with the patient's PSIS, and gently lower your forearm into the space between the three landmarks. Make sure to use a kind elbow, directing pressure with the proximal third of the ulna, not with the olecranon (use your olecranon for reference, not treatment). Lunge down to rest your forearm in this space, treating the multifidus. You can gently lunge back a little to traction the muscles (this is very subtle). The treatment starts off static (just hold). To add movement, turn your forearm between pronation and supination very slowly. Additional movement can come from making a windshield-wiper motion with your forearm (internal and external rotation of the shoulder). As a third option, you can combine pronation and supination with the windshield-wiper motion. Regardless of which option you add to the treatment, keep the proximal third of the ulna in contact with the area. You are not gliding the forearm forward and back or side to side. The treatment stays in one spot.

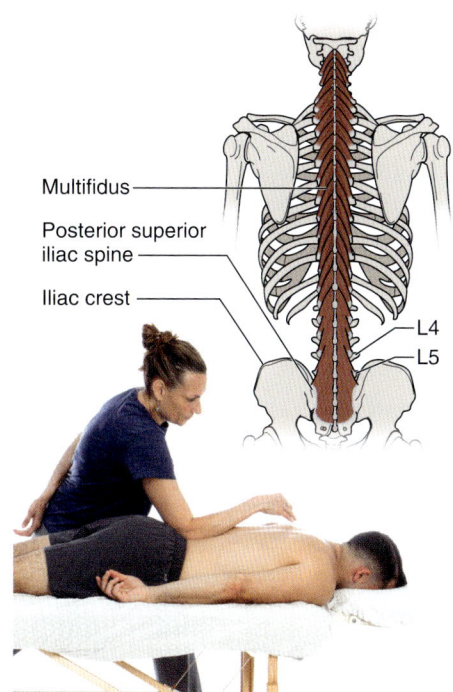

Figure 8.4 For the multifidus treatment, use a kind elbow in the space between the posterior superior iliac spine, the top of the sacrum, and the spinous processes of L4 and L5. Apply pressure with the proximal third of the ulna, not with the tip of the olecranon.

Once you have warmed through the erectors and the multifidus, you can better approach the quadratus lumborum, which sits off the transverse processes between the iliac crest and the 12th rib. From the prone position, you can use a kind elbow in the space between the iliac crest, 12th rib, and transverse processes. However, the space is very small; depending on the size of your forearm, this may not be an effective treatment (you want to especially stay off the 12th rib, because it is floating). As an alternative, you can use your fingertips (make sure your nails are short and clean) or the side-lying position outlined later in this chapter (see the Side-Lying Treatment section), which allows for you to open the space more.

Anterior Abdominal Region

The anterior abdominal region runs from the lower border of the ribs to the pubic bone, extends out to the iliac crest, and wraps around to the thoracolumbar fascia (figure 8.5). The abdominal muscles have bony attachments but also soft tissue attachments, attaching to each other. For this reason, they are subject to the properties of tensegrity, with pull coming from the myofascial tensions.

Rectus Abdominis

Origin
Crest of the pubis

Insertion
Xiphoid process and costal cartilage of ribs 5, 6, and 7

Action
Bilaterally produces flexion of the lumbar spine and posterior pelvic tilt
Unilaterally produces lateral flexion

Innervation
Intercostal nerves

Stressor Considerations

The rectus abdominis has multiple fascial layers associated with it that need to be considered. The right and left sides of the rectus abdominis are separated by the linea alba (white line), and the body of the muscle contains many tendinous inscriptions that give it the separations into segments (creating the washboard abdominal appearance in some lean individuals). As discussed in chapter 1, the tendinous inscriptions serve to shorten the length of the muscle fibers, allowing for more strength in the fibers while retaining the range of motion. However, the areas of change from muscle to connective tissue make the muscle susceptible to strains.

Additionally, the linea alba separates during pregnancy as the abdomen stretches to accommodate the growing fetus and can fail to return to its prepregnancy state, leading to *diastasis rectus* (abdominal separation), which will weaken the

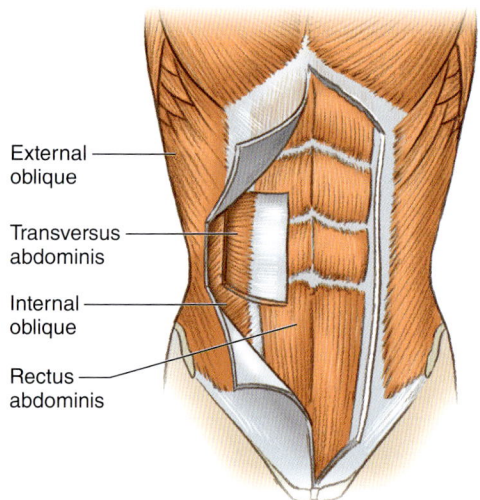

Figure 8.5 The four abdominal muscles have four different fiber directions and four different lines of pull to help create stability in the region, which lacks bony attachments.

muscle and potentially the other abdominal muscles that attach here. Treatment of diastasis rectus is outside the scope of manual therapy, but manual therapy can be used to alleviate associated myofascial pain. If the fascial lines of the rectus abdominis were not enough to lead to dysfunction, the other three abdominal muscles have attachments into the fascia of the rectus abdominis and the linea alba, meaning dysfunction in the other muscles can become a stressor of the rectus abdominis.

External Obliques

Origin
Dovetail with the serratus anterior at the border of the lower eight ribs (ribs 5-12)

Insertion
Anterior half of the iliac crest, inguinal ligament, and pubic crest

Fascia of the rectus abdominis

Action
Bilaterally produce flexion of the lumbar spine and posterior pelvic tilt

Unilaterally produce lateral flexion as well as lumbar rotation to the contralateral side

Innervation
Intercostal nerves

Iliohypogastric nerve

Ilioinguinal nerve

Stressor Considerations
The numerous attachments (origin and insertion) of the external obliques put them in position to have multiple areas of concern. The superior attachment to the ribs near the serratus anterior means there is some involvement with breathing, and compensatory breathing patterns (as outlined in chapter 2) can put stress on the muscle. Distally, the external obliques attach to the inguinal ligament, a connection with the fascia lata, and the rectus abdominus, meaning they are anchored into soft tissue structures with little attachment to bone. The action of contralateral rotation places the external obliques under stress with activities involving rotation. However, remember the anatomical structure: More rotation of the spine occurs in the thoracic region compared with the lumbar region. In addition to the more traditional transverse plane rotation, the external oblique contracts when the shoulder is brought to the opposite hip (involving the muscle on the ipsilateral side of the moving shoulder), a type of rotation that is multiplanar because it involves both rotation and flexion. For activities that involve rotation to one side, such as rotation to the left, the right and left external obliques serve as antagonists to each other. When rotating to the left, the right side is concentrically contracted while the left side is eccentrically contracted. If a conscious effort is not made to strengthen and stretch both sides, the area can be subject to myofascial dysfunction.

Internal Obliques

Origin
Upper half of the inguinal ligament
Anterior two-thirds of the iliac crest and the lumbar fascia

Insertion
Costal cartilage of ribs 8, 9, and 10
Linea alba

Action
Bilaterally produce flexion of the lumbar spine and posterior pelvic tilt
Unilaterally produce lateral flexion, as well as lumbar rotation to the ipsilateral side

Innervation
Intercostal nerves
Iliohypogastric nerve
Ilioinguinal nerve

Stressor Considerations

The internal obliques have an opposite configuration from the external obliques, in which the origin and insertion are reversed. Because of this arrangement, the stressors are similar in relation to being an accessory breathing muscle and in having fascial attachments. The increase in fascial attachments means the muscles are subject to the properties and pulls of tensegrity. For the internal obliques, the muscle fibers run in opposing directions to the external obliques. Therefore, the rotation action is in the opposite direction: When the right internal oblique contracts, the right side rotates (ipsilateral rotation). This action does not change the concept that one side is working concentrically while the other is eccentrically contracted; rather, it just changes the side (right or left) of reference. The advantage of the muscles working in opposition may be that it forces the clinician to work both right and left sides regardless of the action.

Transversus Abdominis

Origin
Lateral third of the inguinal ligament
Internal rim of the iliac crest
Internal surface of the costal cartilage of ribs 7, 8, 9, 10, 11, and 12
Lumbar fascia

Insertion
   Pubic crest
   Abdominal aponeurosis to the linea alba

Function
   Pulls the abdominal wall inward, such as with forced expiration to compress the contents of the abdomen

Innervation
   Intercostal nerves
   Iliohypogastric nerve
   Ilioinguinal nerve

Stressor Considerations

The attachments of the transversus abdominis are lateral to medial, instead of the normal proximal to distal arrangement, and include fascial attachments at both the origin and the insertion. The muscle fibers of the transversus abdominis run horizontal in a direction that is not representative of any actions (the fibers run parallel to the transverse plane). Instead of producing a movement, the transversus abdominis has the function of pulling the abdominal wall inward, creating a back brace of sorts when the muscle is tightened (contracted). Dancers are often taught the importance of engaging the transversus abdominis to hold their postures. Many of the principles of Pilates are centered around engagement of the transversus abdominis. The same principles have been added to rehabilitation principles for those with low back pain. From a treatment perspective, the muscle lies deep to the rest of the abdominal muscles and the thoracolumbar fascia. Direct treatment will occur through the other muscles; therefore, no specific transversus abdominis treatment is given.

Abdomen Supine Treatment

Warming of the abdomen can start with spiraling of the fascia (figure 8.6). With the patient supine, face into the table with your legs in a lunge position, squatting low. Take one of your arms and put it underneath the patient, just above their iliac crest. Bring your arm across their entire back until your fingertips can reach the opposite side of the patient's abdomen. Place your other hand on their near side, with the heel of your hand close to the table (fingers up) (figure 8.6a). Simply stand up in your lunge, simultaneously pulling with your far hand and pushing with your near hand (figure 8.6b). This technique will create a spiral of the fascia and muscles where you are essentially pushing and pulling the muscles around the bones (for additional details, see techniques in chapter 3 and spiraling of the thigh in chapter 9). If the patient requests an increase in pressure, have the patient turn toward you (in the opposite direction of your push). At this point, the patient is in charge of pressure; if it is too much, instruct them to back off. Keep holding the technique to achieve a release. Make sure to direct the patient to release before you let go. You can do this a few times, especially if you need to readjust your hands, but you can stay in the same spot and still affect the fascia of the entire torso.

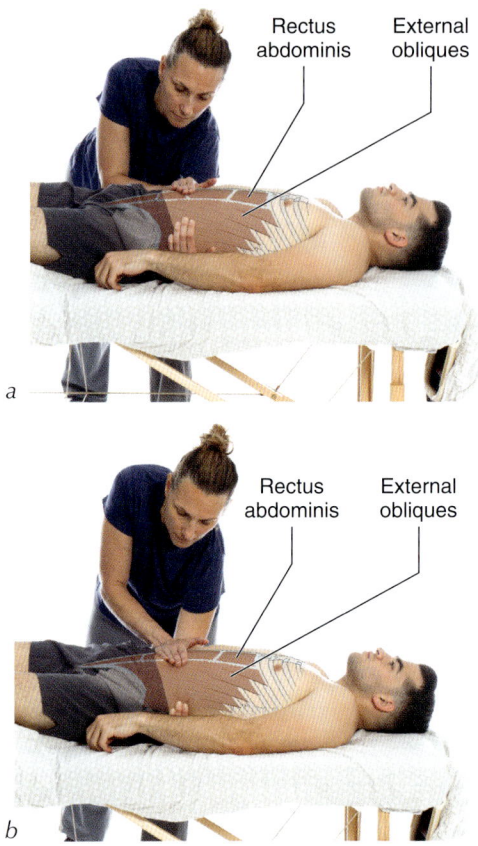

Figure 8.6 *(a)* Spiraling of the abdomen is performed with the clinician placing one hand underneath the client's body to the opposite side of their abdomen and the other hand on the same-side of the abdomen. The clinician starts in a lunge. *(b)* When the clinician stands up, the bottom hand should move toward them as the top hand moves away.

Cautions with Abdominal Spiraling

It is important to note that abdominal spiraling can be used prior to low back treatments as well. However, it is not recommended to perform abdominal spiraling in the prone position. Simply do the treatment supine, and then ask the patient to change to the prone position when it is time for the remainder of the treatment.

Treatment of the rectus abdominis, the most superficial muscle, would follow the spiraling warm-up. To identify the location and width of the muscle, simply have the patient lift their head off the table to engage the muscle fibers. Doing so will allow you to see how wide to place your hands. Using both hands, grasp the sides of the rectus abdominis for the lift and shift technique (figure 8.7). Start by simply lifting the muscle and holding. Remind the patient to breathe (this is a good reminder for you too). As the fascia starts to become more compliant, you can slowly traction off the pubic bone (traction superiorly, toward the head) or off the xiphoid process and ribs with a slow traction inferiorly. The muscle can also be moved medially and laterally. Depending on the size of your hands and the size of the muscle, you can work bilaterally (both the right and left rectus abdominis) or unilaterally (right or left side, splitting the muscle at the level of the linea alba).

Treatment of the oblique muscle bellies is best done with the patient in a side-lying position and will be outlined in the next section. The fascial attachments of the obliques and the transversus abdominis are treated with this approach as well as with spiraling. The transversus abdominis is only treated through the other muscles.

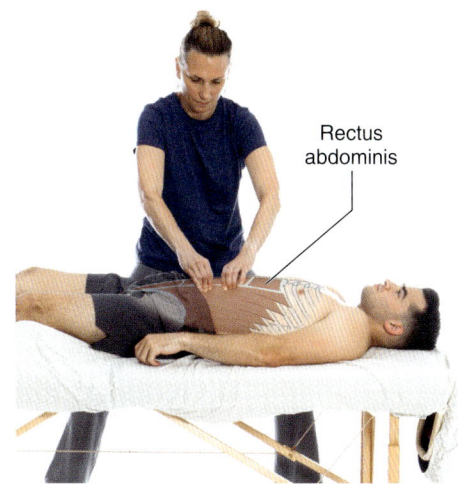

Figure 8.7 The rectus abdominis is grasped in both hands (right and left side muscles) for the lift and shift technique. The muscle can be moved superiorly and inferiorly or medially and laterally to complete the treatment.

Side-Lying Treatment

Warming prior to the side-lying treatment should be done with the patient in either a prone or supine position, depending on your preference and the muscles being addressed. Make sure to consider the size of your patient prior to the treatment, because they will be taller in the side-lying position than when they are prone or supine. It is best to start with a lower table for warming rather than to strain when you change the patient to a side-lying position (i.e., working lower is always better than working higher). If your table cannot be lowered, consider using a stationary stool to stand on if you can balance effectively.

To address the quadratus lumborum with the patient in the side-lying position (continued from the prone treatment), start with warming the tissue prone. When you get to the last step of treating the quadratus lumborum, then place the patient in a side-lying position, with the treatment side facing up toward the ceiling. Stand behind the patient. Instruct the patient to come closer to the table edge where you are positioned, monitoring them so they do not fall off the table (I like to stand at the edge of the table so I create a barrier preventing them from going too far, but you can also use a hand to guide them because they are not facing the table edge). The patient can rest their head either on their own arm or a pillow if available. The patient should stack their legs one on top of another, if comfortable. If that is not comfortable, you may place a pillow or bolster under the top leg and have the bottom leg comfortably forward on the table. However, this position opens the space between the 12th rib and the iliac crest, so avoid using something that is too high here.

Stand in a lunge position facing into the table (one leg in front of the other). Using the proximal third of your forearm, gently rest in the space between the 12th rib, iliac crest, and transverse processes, just off the erector spinae (figure 8.8). (*Note:* Do not push down from the top; engage from the side facing you.) The treatment is a simple static hold at first. To add to the treatment, have the patient slowly and gently drop their top leg off the table behind them. (Here is where positioning is key: If the patient is in the right spot, the leg will drop without them falling and with you behind as a barrier. If they are too close to the edge, they may not be balanced properly.) If you need to help them, use your free hand (ideally, the one closest to their feet) to help guide them. If the patient's muscles are very tight, they will not be able to move the leg far. As an alternative, they can also reach their same-side (top) arm above their head to open the space. Despite the setup and all the steps needed, this treatment does not take long and is very effective.

For the abdominal muscles, the manual therapy treatment will use the same principles. Make sure to warm the abdominal region first. For the first half of the treatment, you will use the same patient setup: Place the patient in a side-lying position with the treatment side facing up. You are behind the patient, with the patient close to the edge of the table but still supported. The patient's legs can be stacked or bolstered. Their head should be supported with either the arm or a pillow. You should be facing into the table in a lunge position. The proximal third of your forearm will be used, but the positioning will be more anterior (figure 8.9b). The elbow can be open to approximately 75 degrees of flexion, resting on the obliques,

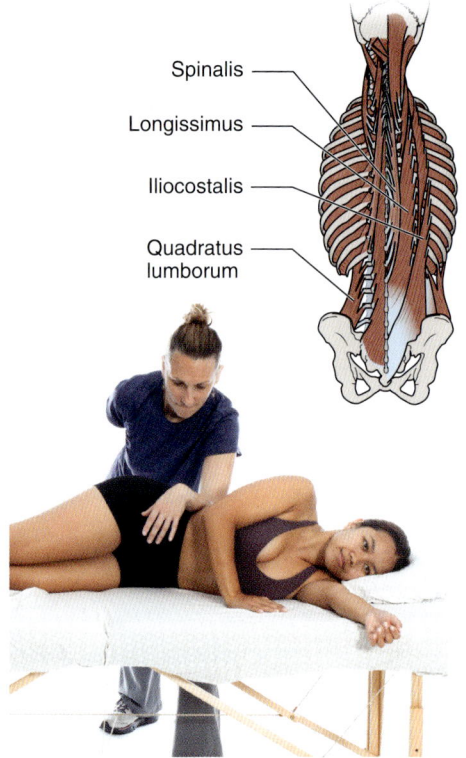

Figure 8.8 Side-lying treatment allows the space between the 12th rib and the iliac crest to open for working on the quadratus lumborum. To create more of a stretch, the patient can drop their top leg behind them or reach out with their arm.

just medial to the midline of the side of the body. The treatment is an engagement into the external obliques with a gentle traction toward the table at an approximately 45- to 60-degree angle (not straight down to the table and not straight across the body, but somewhere in between). Think of working along the muscle, as opposed to down into the muscle. To increase the engagement, have the patient lift their top arm up and back, rotating toward you (and away from the point of engagement of the muscles). Doing so will create a stretch of the external obliques (remember, they are contralateral rotators).

To treat the internal obliques, simply switch your position to face the patient, and have the patient move toward the other side of the table (you are still working the side that is up). The treatment is similar but from the other side. Use the same lunge into the table and the same aspect of your forearm. Here, you are working posteriorly to the midline of the side of the body at the same angle (figure 8.9a). Have the patient use their top arm to reach toward you, rotating toward you and away from the traction of the forearm (remember, the internal obliques perform ipsilateral rotation, so they are lengthened in this position). Because the internal obliques lie deep to the external obliques, the external obliques should be treated first.

When ending any of the treatments just described, remember to exit the treatment with care and ease. Just as you engage slowly, you want to reverse the movement slowly and cautiously. Always make sure the patient has returned from their movements before releasing your hold.

Chapter 8 Lower Back and Abdomen

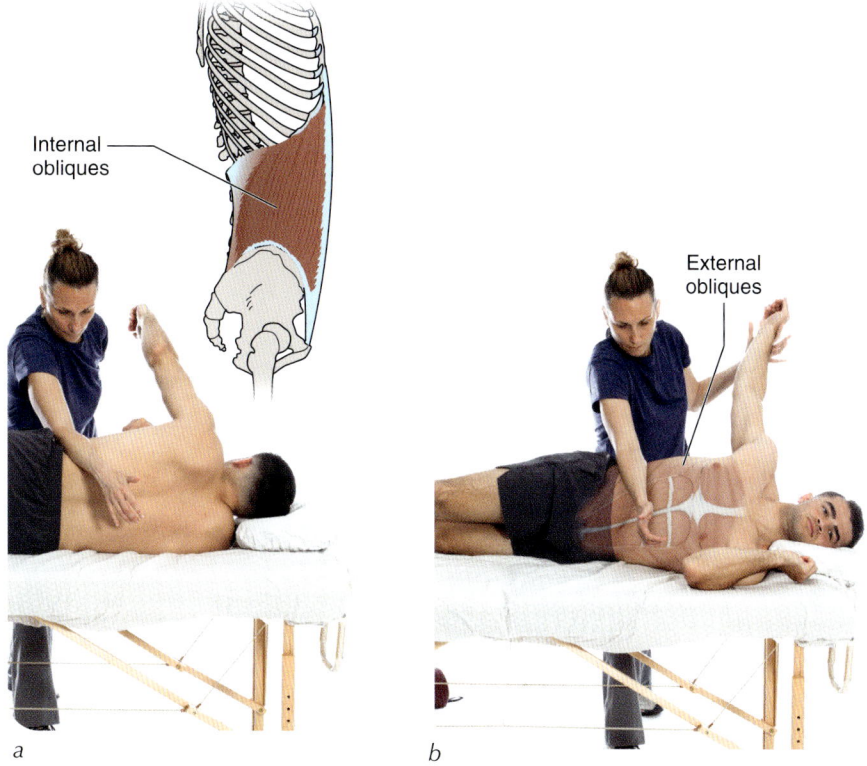

Figure 8.9 *(a)* The clinician is positioned facing the patient. While the clinician engages the tissue to the posterior aspect of the body, the patient can rotate toward the clinician to create more pressure. *(b)* To treat the external obliques, simply face the other way.

WHY DOES THE CLINICIAN CARE?

Low back pain is a common complaint among all active individuals and many nonactive individuals as well. Most back issues are related to muscular imbalance. This imbalance can be caused by poor posture and disruption of the natural alignment of the spine, but it can also be caused by the stress that sport places on the muscles and spine. As pointed out in the beginning of this chapter, the muscles in this area have few bony attachments and rely on the tensegrity of the myofascial structures. The most likely causes of back pain and the ability of manual therapy to address them make for a perfect match. Remember to include some stretching and strengthening (if within the scope of practice) to keep the body ready for activity.

Hip, Thigh, and Knee

From a sport perspective, change in direction for the lower body is initiated by the hips. For example, a basketball coach tells defenders to watch the waist of the player they are guarding to see if they are going to drive right, left, or straight. A football coach tells the defensive backs to watch the hips to see the direction of travel of the wide receiver they are covering. In anatomy, joint movements are discussed from distal to proximal, where hip flexion is the action of lifting the leg (*flexion* is defined as a decrease in the joint angle). From a functional perspective, hip flexion is the action of sitting down with the feet on the floor so the pelvis moves closer to the feet. Instead of the origin moving toward the insertion, the insertion remains stable and the origin moves. Considering how the body moves, as opposed to how the anatomy is taught, will help the clinician prepare the appropriate treatment for the hip, thigh, and knee, including manual therapy and strengthening.

Joint Structure

In examining the structure of the hip, similarity is seen between the hip and the shoulder. In the hip, the pelvic girdle supports the lower extremity; in the shoulder, the shoulder (pectoral) girdle supports the upper extremity. Both girdles attach to the axial skeleton: the ilium to the sacrum for the hip, and the clavicle to the sternum for the shoulder. The series of joints in the hip, however, follow a more traditional anatomical structure with three joints: the pubic symphysis (one joint located at the midline), the sacroiliac joint (one left and one right), and the acetabulofemoral joint (one left and one right).

Sacroiliac Joint

The *sacroiliac joint* is a gliding joint where the sacrum meets with the ilium, one of the three fused bones of the coxal bone (ilium, ischium, and pubic bones). Essentially, the sacrum is wedged between the posterior aspect of the coxal bones. The joint does not produce actions; movement is gliding and subtle as the joint has very strong ligamentous support that prevents movement in any of the planes.

The strong ligament structure of the sacroiliac joint spans the anterior and posterior surfaces, preventing motion and providing stability to the pelvis. There are two accessory ligaments: the sacrotuberous ligament (from the sacrum to the ischial tuberosity) and the sacrospinous ligament (from the sacrum to the ischial spine). Both ligaments aid in stabilizing the joint, preventing it from tipping forward. Additionally, the ligaments create the greater and lesser sciatic foramen and serve as muscle attachments.

Pubic Symphysis

The right and left pubic bones meet each other anteriorly to form the *pubic symphysis*. Sitting between the two bones is a fibrocartilage disc. The pubic symphysis is not a synovial joint; rather, it is a fibrocartilaginous joint that provides no movement and does not act in any planes. The exception to the no-movement rule is during the latter stages of pregnancy, when the hormone relaxin is released to allow for opening of the birth canal. Although this is a book on sports massage, keep in mind there are athletes training through pregnancy and returning to sport following childbirth. Therefore, pregnancy may influence this joint and the muscles that attach around the pubic bone, including the rectus abdominis.

Acetabulofemoral Joint

The *acetabulofemoral joint* is the articulation of the head of the femur in the acetabulum to create a ball-and-socket joint. The acetabulum is a depression in the coxal bone where the ilium, ischium, and pubic bones meet and eventually fuse. Unlike the glenoid fossa of the shoulder, the acetabulum is a very deep bony depression that, in normal bone formation, can fit more than half of the head of the femur. There is a labrum here, too, that attaches to the edges of the acetabulum, providing even more depth to the structure. The hip joint is relatively stable with movement in all planes.

LIGAMENTS

The capsule of the hip is very strong and is supported by three ligaments, each named for its bony attachments. The *iliofemoral ligament* runs from the anterior superior iliac spine (ASIS) to the lesser and greater trochanters. This ligament aids in trunk stabilization and upright gait. The *ischiofemoral ligament* is the weakest of the three ligaments, running from the posterior rim of the acetabulum at the ischium, spiraling up to the greater trochanter. The *pubofemoral ligament*, running from the pubic ramus and acetabular rim to the intertrochanteric fossa, reinforces the medial joint capsule and prevents excessive abduction.

ACETABULUM AND LABRUM

The labrum provides depth to the acetabulum and, just like in the shoulder, can be injured. Labral tears in the hip create a structural change, often causing pain and limiting range of motion. In addition, the acetabulum can vary in size: It can be shallow (dysplastic), which may increase the risk of hip dislocation, or deep (pincer), where there is just a deeper socket or the presence of bony overgrowth. Surgery to the hip, whether open or arthroscopic, can disrupt the joint capsule, which serves as an attachment for the rectus femoris (as discussed later in this chapter). Manual therapy to the hip and thigh can relieve many symptoms of conditions affecting the joint, but it cannot treat the injury itself.

Thigh

The thigh is included here because much of the manual therapy treatment involves the muscles of the thigh and the fascia lata. The fascia lata (discussed in chapter 1) surrounds the thigh and is continuous with the fascial structures above and below. The inguinal ligament found running from the pubic tubercle to the ASIS is the superior gathering of the fascia lata, whereas the iliotibial band is the distal gathering near the knee. The muscles of the thigh are divided into three compartments: anterior (quadriceps group), posterior (hamstring group), and medial (adductor group). The musculature on the lateral thigh is the vastus lateralis, part of the quadriceps group. The abductors of the hip are located on the lateral aspect of the ilium, not on the thigh. In addition, the quadriceps group and the hamstring group provide knee extension and flexion, respectively. Therefore, it is important to consider these muscles, as well as those noted later in the Muscles section, for their implication in knee pain.

Knee Joint and Patellofemoral Joint

The knee joint proper is a modified hinge joint in which the condyles of the femur rest on the tibial plateau. Flexion and extension are the common actions associated with the knee; however, the knee also allows for movement in the transverse planes, with internal and external rotation being controlled by the hamstring group and the popliteus. The knee is supported by a strong capsule, intracapsular ligaments, and extracapsular ligaments, as well as the patella and the associated musculature. To accommodate the rounded femoral condyles, two menisci (medial and lateral) sitting on the tibial plateau assist in joint function as well as shock absorption. Knee joint function is optimized with full range of motion, particularly extension that may have a lag secondary to the response of the distal hamstrings to stress. As a postural muscle, the distal hamstrings respond to stress by shortening and, per Davis' law, there is a loss of tissue to maintain the appropriate relationship of the muscle to the insertion distal to the knee joint. Additionally, arthrogenic inhibition may occur after knee injury and surgery, limiting the firing of the quadriceps group as a protective measure (Houglum 2016). For example, a patient with an extension lag can benefit from treatment to the distal hamstrings, whereas a client with arthrogenic inhibition can benefit from treatment to the quadriceps group. Because there is a strong overlap between the muscles that act on the hip and knee, there is little need for a knee-only chapter in this book; the manual therapy treatments are best presented here.

LIGAMENTS

The knee has four main ligaments: the intracapsular cruciate ligaments, the capsular medial collateral ligament, and the extracapsular lateral collateral ligament. The anterior and posterior cruciate ligaments assist in rotational stability as well as anterior and posterior translation of the tibia on the femur, respectively. The medial collateral ligament features two layers and is part of the medial joint capsule. There is also a connection of the deep layer of the medial collateral to the medial meniscus, often resulting in both structures being injured together. The lateral collateral ligament is extracapsular, sitting outside the lateral joint capsule as it runs from the lateral femoral condyle to the head of the fibula. Although injuries and any subsequent surgical repair of the ligaments are outside the scope of this text, individual muscle treatments addressed in this chapter are important for clinicians to consider when a patient is rehabilitating and recovering from an injury.

MENISCI

The medial and lateral menisci sit on the tibial plateau and help to provide a better fit for the femoral condyles. The medial meniscus has more of a C shape, whereas the lateral meniscus has a more closed U shape. The medial meniscus is more firmly attached to the tibia, which, along with its attachment to the medial collateral ligament, makes it more prone to injury. The lateral meniscus moves more freely, making it less likely to be injured acutely. Based on their role in absorbing forces, both menisci can be injured in a more chronic or overuse scenario.

Patellofemoral Joint

The patella is a sesamoid bone, embedded in the quadriceps tendon. Although the patella gives the quadriceps increased mechanical efficiency, it also provides bony protection to the anterior aspect of the knee and absorbs and transmits forces through the joint's articular surfaces. During knee flexion and extension, the patella moves through the femoral groove. The vastus medialis and the vastus lateralis control the medial and lateral pull of the patella, respectively. Because of its presence in the quadriceps tendon, the patella is subjected to the dysfunctions that may occur in the vastus medialis and the vastus lateralis. Typically, it is the larger, stronger vastus lateralis that influences the pull of the patella more laterally.

MUSCLES OF THE HIP AND THIGH

The attachments of the muscles in this chapter span from the ilium, above the hip joint, to the tibia and the fibula, below the knee joint. Treatments for these muscles can be used for issues that may present at the hip, sacroiliac joint, pubic symphysis, and knee. Although the individual muscles are listed by their location and attachments, most of the treatments can be streamlined into anterior, lateral, and posterior treatments. Although the adductors can be treated with the patient in a side-lying position, they do very well in a figure-four position in which the hip is externally rotated, allowing for the medial aspect of the thigh to face up. It is important to maintain boundaries when working on muscles that attach close to the genitalia; therefore, considerations are made for working respectfully in the pelvic region.

Quadriceps Group

The four muscles on the anterior thigh make up the quadriceps group. The rectus femoris is the only one of the four muscles that crosses the hip, thus acting in hip flexion (figure 9.1). The three vastus muscles are located on the femur and cross the knee (tibiofemoral joint). All four muscles come together distally to form the quadriceps tendon, which surrounds the patella, ultimately inserting on the tibial tuberosity via the patellar tendon. The medial and lateral pull of the patella, embedded in the quadriceps tendon, is controlled by the vastus lateralis and the vastus medialis. The quadriceps group has the concentric action of knee flexion and is responsible for eccentric action during deceleration. For example, when a person is landing from a jump or decelerating from a sprint, the quadriceps group is responsible for slowing the body down. In addition, the quadriceps is an antigravity muscle, working to control descent when changing levels, such as when descending stairs. As mentioned in chapter 4, the quadriceps group can become inhibited and often suffers from atrophy in association with knee injuries and surgeries.

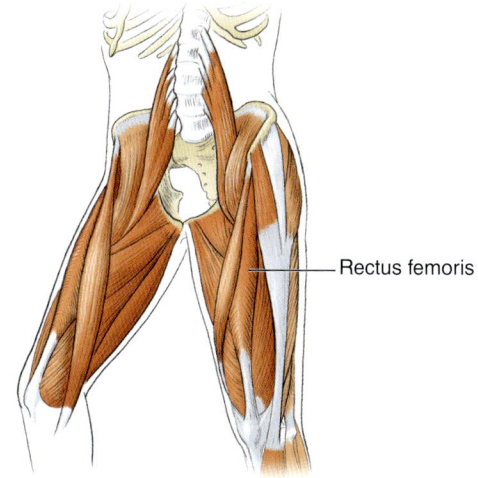

Rectus Femoris

Origin
- Anterior inferior iliac spine
- Slip that attaches to the groove above the acetabulum as well as the capsule of the hip

Figure 9.1 The rectus femoris crosses the hip and the knee with a slip of the origin attaching to the acetabulum as well as the anterior inferior iliac spine. The four vastus muscles only cross the knee, acting in knee extension. The vastus lateralis and the vastus medialis contribute to keeping the patella tracking correctly.

Insertion
  Superior aspect of the patella and patellar tendon to the tibial tuberosity

Action
  Flexion of the hip (acetabulofemoral joint)
  Extension of the knee (tibiofemoral joint); also contributes to anterior rotation of the pelvis

Innervation
  Femoral nerve

Stressor Considerations

As a two-jointed muscle, the rectus femoris is stressed differently proximally and distally. Proximally, the muscle tends to be more postural—shortening, tightening, and contracting. It is not uncommon for the rectus femoris to contribute to tight hip flexors and an anteriorly rotated pelvis. Distally, the four quadriceps are apt to be phasic, lengthened, and weakened. Additionally, the slip of the rectus femoris that attaches to the acetabulum may be affected by surgery to the hip joint, including labral pathology, causing scar tissue to develop in the area. When treating the rectus femoris, the clinician is advised to provide care to both the hip flexors and the anterior thigh regardless of which area is causing the issue.

Vastus Lateralis

Origin
  Intertrochanteric line
  Anterior and inferior border of the greater trochanter
  Gluteal tuberosity
  Upper half of the linea aspera and lateral intermuscular septum

Insertion
  Lateral border of the patella and patellar tendon to the tibial tuberosity

Action
  Extension of the knee (tibiofemoral joint)
  Functions with the vastus medialis to keep the patella within the femoral groove

Innervation
  Femoral nerve

Stressor Considerations

The vastus lateralis is the largest of the vastus muscles, comprising 40 percent of the cross-sectional area of the quadriceps. Inherently, the vastus lateralis is stronger than the vastus medialis, with which it works to keep the patella gliding in the femoral groove. Therefore, with patellofemoral dysfunction, the larger, stronger vastus lateralis often pulls the patella laterally. Additionally, the lateral intermuscular septum is part of the vast origin of the vastus lateralis. This connective tissue attachment, which is shared with the biceps femoris of the hamstring group, can influence the pull of the muscle. Finally, the iliotibial band, the lateral overlap of the fascia lata of the thigh, is superficial to the lateral aspect of the vastus lateralis belly. Tightness in the iliotibial band can lead to dysfunction in the vastus lateralis and vice versa.

Vastus Medialis

Origin
Length of the linea aspera on the posterior femur
Medial condylar ridge of the femur

Insertion
Medial half of the upper border of the patella and patellar tendon to the tibial tuberosity

Action
Extension of the knee (tibiofemoral joint)
Functions with the vastus lateralis to maintain the patella in the femoral groove

Innervation
Femoral nerve

Stressor Considerations

The vastus medialis make up 25 percent of the cross-sectional area of the quadriceps group. Medial pull of the patella is initiated by the oblique portion of the muscle, the vastus medialis obliques, which are weak in much of the population but can be well developed in athletes who play soccer (or football, to those not in the United States), in which the kicking motion is prevalent. Based on the size difference between the vastus medialis and the vastus lateralis and the propensity of the vastus medialis toward being weaker while the vastus lateralis tends to be tighter, dysfunction at the patellofemoral joint is often attributed to the weaker vastus medialis. Although strengthening a weaker muscle is always advised, allowing for a release of the lateral structures can also help encourage the vastus medialis to do its job.

Vastus Intermedius

Origin
Upper two-thirds of the anterior surface of the femur

Insertion
Superior border of the patella and patellar tendon to the tibial tuberosity

Action
Extension of the knee (tibiofemoral joint)

Innervation
Femoral nerve

> **Stressor Considerations**
>
> The vastus intermedius lies deep to the rectus femoris. The vastus intermedius is typically not implicated in any issues on its own; therefore, it is typically treated along with the rest of the musculature.

Hamstring Group

Found on the posterior aspect of the thigh, the hamstring group is responsible for hip extension and knee flexion (figure 9.2). The hamstring group is in opposition to the quadriceps group in its actions as well as in its makeup. Whereas the quadriceps group has only one muscle that crosses two joints, all three muscles in the hamstring group cross two joints: The short head of the biceps femoris is the lone muscle that only crosses the knee joint. The hip extensor portion is more phasic in nature, lengthened and weakened; the knee flexor portion is more postural, shortening in response to stress. The quadriceps group functions in deceleration, whereas the hamstring group functions in acceleration. In addition, as the quadriceps contract to produce knee extension, the hamstrings work to control the pelvis by initiating a posterior pelvic tilt. The medial hamstrings (semitendinosus and semimembranosus) are responsible for internal or medial rotation of the knee (occurring when the knee is in flexion), and the biceps femoris, the lateral hamstring, is responsible for external or lateral rotation of the knee.

Present in the hamstrings are various tendinous inscriptions. As outlined in chapter 1, the muscle fibers run from origin to insertion; in some muscles, the muscle belly has connective tissue attachments (tendinous inscriptions) that serve to shorten the muscle fibers, allowing for increased strength while still achieving a greater range of motion than a shorter muscle. However, recall from chapter 4 that muscle strains are more common at the musculotendinous junction, where the muscle tissue meets the connective tissue. The tendinous inscriptions place this change in tissue type in the muscle belly, meaning the hamstring strains occurring in the muscle belly may be at these tendinous inscriptions.

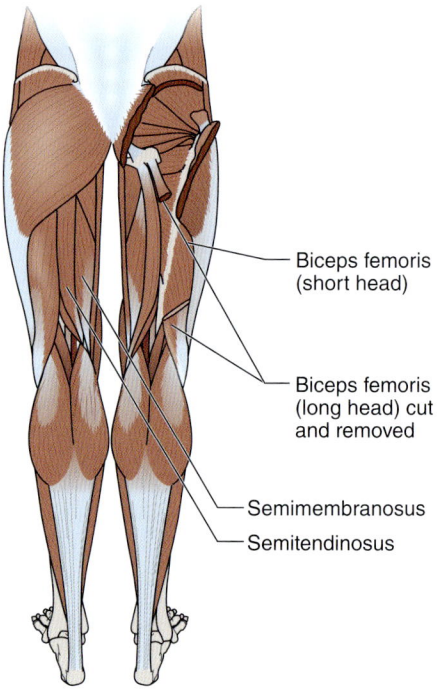

Figure 9.2 The hamstring group from a posterior view. The semitendinosus and the semimembranosus are medial and the biceps femoris is lateral.

Semimembranosus

Origin
  Ischial tuberosity

Insertion
  Posterior medial surface of the medial tibial condyle

Action
  Extension of the hip (acetabulofemoral joint)
  Flexion of the knee (tibiofemoral joint)
  Internal rotation of the flexed knee (tibiofemoral joint)

Innervation
  Tibial nerve

Stressor Considerations

  The origin of the semimembranosus at the ischial tuberosity sits deep to the common attachment of the semitendinosus and the biceps femoris. The name *semimembranosus* is given because the muscle is more membranous at the proximal attachment, with more of the muscle belly found closer to the distal attachment. When palpating for the muscle near its insertion at the posteromedial aspect of the tibia, it is more lateral and flatter than the more medial and rope-like semitendinosus.

Semitendinosus

Origin
  Ischial tuberosity with the tendon of the long head of the biceps femoris

Insertion
  Upper medial surface of the tibia below the medial condyle as part of the pes anserine group with the sartorius and the gracilis

Action
  Extension of the hip (acetabulofemoral joint)
  Flexion of the knee (tibiofemoral joint)
  Internal rotation of the flexed knee (tibiofemoral joint)

Innervation
  Tibial nerve

Stressor Considerations

  The semitendinosus and the biceps femoris share a common origin at the ischial tuberosity. Therefore, treatment of both the medial and lateral aspects of the hamstrings is warranted if there are any concerns at the proximal tendon of either muscle. The semitendinosus has a shorter tendon proximally and a more rope-like tendon distally, which can be found on the medial aspect of the popliteal space. The semitendinosus shares its insertion as well, this time with the gracilis and the sartorius at the pes anserine tendon. There is a bursa associated with the pes anserine attachment; therefore, be cautious with treatment to the insertion if inflammation is present. In the case of bursitis, it would be appropriate to work the three muscle bellies, avoiding the tendon, to help relieve any myofascial restrictions that may be causing the bursitis or preventing effective relief with treatment and rehabilitation.

Biceps Femoris

The biceps femoris is a two-headed muscle on the lateral aspect of the thigh. The long head crosses both the hip and knee joints, whereas the short head only crosses the knee; therefore, it is solely a knee flexor. Interestingly, the two heads have different innervations: the tibial nerve for the long head, as well as the semitendinosus and the semimembranosus, and the common peroneal nerve for the short head. Although both nerves branch from the sciatic nerve, having different innervations is a protective mechanism for the muscle, allowing for knee flexion to occur even if there is damage to one of the nerves.

Long Head

Origin
　Ischial tuberosity with the semitendinosus

Insertion
　Head of the fibula
　Lateral condyle of the tibia

Action
　Extension of the hip (acetabulofemoral joint)
　Flexion of the knee (tibiofemoral joint)
　External rotation of the flexed knee (tibiofemoral joint)

Innervation
　Tibial nerve

Short Head

Origin
　Lower half of the linea aspera
　Lateral condylar ridge of the femur

Insertion
　Head of the fibula
　Lateral condyle of the tibia

Chapter 9 Hip, Thigh, and Knee

Action
Flexion of the knee (tibiofemoral joint)
External rotation of the flexed knee (tibiofemoral joint)

Innervation
Common peroneal nerve

Stressor Considerations

The biceps femoris (long head) shares an origin with the semitendinosus, making treatment of both muscles appropriate for any issues at the proximal attachment. The short head does not cross the hip, making it more efficient in knee flexion than the other three aspects of the hamstrings. If there is pain in the lateral hamstrings without hip extension, it is important to treat the short head of the muscle, focusing on the lateral aspect of the linea aspera, where the muscle originates. Both heads join to form the distal tendon, which inserts at the head of the fibula where the peroneus longus originates (see chapter 10) and is palpable posterior to the iliotibial band. Treatment at the distal tendon should include lateral aspects of both the femur and fibula for effective treatment.

Adductors

The adductor muscles make up the medial portion of the thigh, originating around the pubic rami and the anterior aspect of the ischium to the ischial tuberosity (figure 9.3). Insertion of the muscles spans the posteromedial aspect of the femur from the pectineal line down the length of the linea aspera to the adductor tubercle (for the adductor magnus) and crossing the knee to the pes anserine attachment (for the gracilis). The adductor magnus, the largest of the muscles, sits the most posteriorly, with the rest of the adductors resting on top, as though the adductor magnus is a tray holding up the rest of the muscles. It is important to remember when working with these muscles that the attachments at the pubic bone sit three-dimensionally, meaning the line of pull is not straight medial but always a little anterior or posterior to the femur. The hip adductors are typically phasic and weaker than the hip abductors.

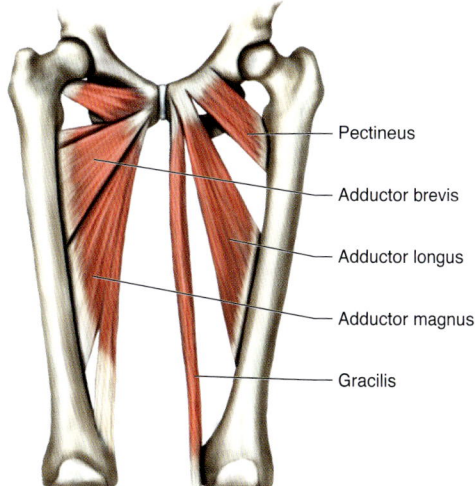

Figure 9.3 The adductor muscles run from the pubic and ischial bones to the femur, except for the gracilis, which crosses the knee, inserting with the pes anserine group on the tibia.

Pectineus

Origin
Anterior surface of the pubis just above the pubic crest

Insertion
Pectineal line from the lesser trochanter to the linea aspera

Action
Flexion of the hip (acetabulofemoral joint)
Adduction of the hip (acetabulofemoral joint)
External rotation of the hip (acetabulofemoral joint)

Innervation
Femoral nerve

Stressor Considerations

The pectineus is sometimes placed with the adductor group and sometimes with the anterior hip muscles, sharing characteristics of both. It also makes up the floor of the femoral triangle of the hip. Although the pectineus is typically innervated by the femoral nerve, which is responsible for the anterior thigh muscles, a variation has it innervated by the obturator nerve, which is responsible for the adductors (less than 10 percent of cases). From a stressor standpoint, the pectineus may be associated with the hip flexors, postural muscles that respond to stress by shortening, or with the adductors, which are phasic and respond to stress by weakening. This is an example of muscles adopting a different pattern based on the stresses placed on it (as discussed in chapter 1). Although the pectineus is typically not treated in isolation, the muscle should be considered with treatment of either the hip adductors or hip flexors, especially in sports that use adduction and hip flexion, such as ice hockey.

Adductor Longus

Origin
Anterior surface of the superior ramus of the pubis just below the crest

Insertion
Middle one-third of the linea aspera

Action
Adduction of the hip (acetabulofemoral joint)
Assists in hip flexion (acetabulofemoral joint)

Innervation
Obturator nerve

Stressor Considerations

The adductor longus is typically phasic, responding to stress by lengthening and weakening. This muscle sits more anteriorly than the rest of the adductors (except the pectineus), and it makes up the lateral aspect of the floor of the femoral triangle (sitting medial to the pectineus).

Adductor Brevis

Origin
Anterior surface of the inferior pubic ramus

Insertion
Lower two-thirds of the pectineal line
Upper half of the medial lip of the linea aspera

Action
Adduction of the hip (acetabulofemoral joint) and external rotation of the hip (acetabulofemoral joint)
Assists in hip flexion (acetabulofemoral joint)

Innervation
Obturator nerve

Stressor Considerations

The adductor brevis originates on the inferior pubic ramus, causing it to sit more posteriorly on the pubic bone (from a three-dimensional perspective). The adductor brevis inserts between the pectineus and adductor longus on the pectineal line and the linea aspera; the three muscles insert on the femur from proximal to distal in the following order: pectineus, adductor brevis, adductor longus. Like the rest of the adductor group, the adductor brevis is also a phasic muscle.

Adductor Magnus

Origin
Pubic ramus
Ischial ramus
Ischial tuberosity

Insertion
On the femur at the linea aspera, medial condylar ridge, and adductor tubercle

Action
Adduction of the hip
Extension of the hip
External rotation of the hip (acetabulofemoral joint)

Innervation
    Mostly obturator nerve

    Hamstring portion by the tibial nerve

Stressor Considerations

The adductor magnus is the largest, and thus the strongest, of the adductor muscles. It sits the most posteriorly, having a fascial attachment to the semimembranosus, the deepest of the hamstring group. Because of this fascial attachment, its origin reaching to the ischial tuberosity, and its contribution to hip extension, the adductor magnus is sometimes called the *fourth hamstring*. However, it does not cross the knee and has no role in knee flexion (Travell and Simons 1983). The adductor magnus also has an adductor hiatus, a space between the muscle bellies allowing the femoral artery and vein to traverse from anterior to posterior into the popliteal space. The adductor magnus is the most complex of the adductors, making it the most likely focus of the manual therapy treatment.

Gracilis

Origin
    Anteromedial edge of the descending ramus of the pubis near the pubic symphysis

Insertion
    Upper medial surface of the tibia below the medial condyle as part of the pes anserine group with the sartorius and the semitendinosus

Action
    Adduction of the hip (acetabulofemoral joint)

    Assists with hip flexion and hip internal rotation (acetabulofemoral joint) and weak knee flexion (tibiofemoral joint)

Innervation
    Obturator nerve

Stressor Considerations

The gracilis originates close to the pubic symphysis with a very short tendon, meaning the musculotendinous junction is very close to the pubic bone. Since the musculotendinous junction is the location common to muscle strains, strains of the gracilis will appear close to the bone, perhaps mimicking *osteitis pubis* (inflammation of the pubic bone) or resulting in an *avulsion fracture* (the tendon pulling from the bone at the site of the injury). The belly of the gracilis is medial to the rest of the adductors. It runs from the pubic bone to the tibia with no attachments to the femur. Distally, the gracilis becomes part of the pes anserine group with the sartorius and semitendinosus and is the only adductor to cross the knee, thus acting on the knee joint in producing flexion. As with the other adductors, the gracilis is phasic, responding to stress by shortening and lengthening.

Thigh Treatment

To warm the thigh, start with one of the most versatile myofascial treatments, spiraling of the thigh, which serves to release the fascia in all three thigh compartments (figure 9.4). The treatment is done with the patient in the supine position. Face into the table while maintaining a low lunge position. Reach one of your hands under the patient's thigh and rest your hand as far medially and superiorly as possible (a somewhat uncomfortable position to start). Place your other hand inferiorly on the lateral aspect of the patient's thigh (see figure 9.4a). Spiraling is achieved by simply standing up in the lunge, causing the medial hand to move more inferiorly and the lateral hand to move more superiorly (see figure 9.4b). The muscles and fascia of the thigh internally rotate around the femur. To add more pressure to the treatment, instruct the patient to actively externally rotate from the hip (I simply tell the patient, "Turn your leg toward me," because most people on the table will not know what it means to externally rotate the hip). The patient is now in charge of their own pressure. If they would like more pressure, they can rotate more; if they need less pressure, you can simply tell them to back off. Hold the position to allow the fascia to release.

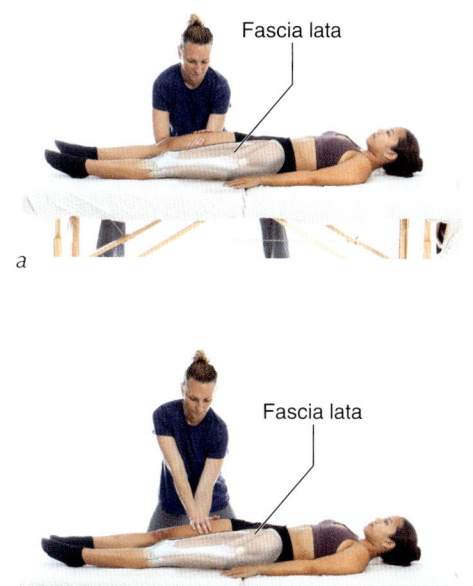

Figure 9.4 *(a)* The start of the spiral begins with the therapist in a low lunge; one hand reaches under the leg to the superomedial portion of the thigh, while the near hand begins near the inferolateral portion. *(b)* The actual treatment begins when the therapist stands up out of the lunge, rotating the muscles of the thigh around the femur.

Before you end the technique or if you are taking a break, make sure to have the patient relax (release the rotation) prior to disengaging from the fascia. If you need to readjust your hands, use the same process for disengagement prior to readjusting your hands. There is no need to move more inferiorly or superiorly with this technique; regardless of where you start, you will affect all the muscle attaching to or crossing through the thigh.

Anterior Thigh

Treatment of the anterior thigh can continue with glides along the anterior femur to address the quadriceps group. Because of the large surface area, any of your tools can be used to perform the glides, such as a loose fist (which keeps the wrist more neutral), the heel of the hand, or even the proximal third of the ulna of the forearm for a larger surface area (make sure not to bend the elbow too much, and not to use the olecranon). Glides performed more medially will address the vastus medialis, especially near the medial aspect of the patella. After the glides, the rectus femoris may have had enough restrictions released to allow for lifting and shifting of the distal aspect off the superior border of the patella (the proximal aspect will be addressed with the anterior hip treatment) (figure 9.5). Because the vastus intermedius is deep to the rectus femoris, there is not a different treatment to address the muscle. Glides through the rectus femoris may address any concerns, and lifting the rectus femoris will address the fascial connection between the two muscles (deep to the rectus femoris and superficial to the vastus intermedius). The vastus lateralis can be treated with glides along the superolateral surface of the anterior thigh. Additionally, you will learn how to position the patient laterally later in this chapter (see the Treatment of the Anterior and Lateral Hip section), which will further address the vastus lateralis under the iliotibial band.

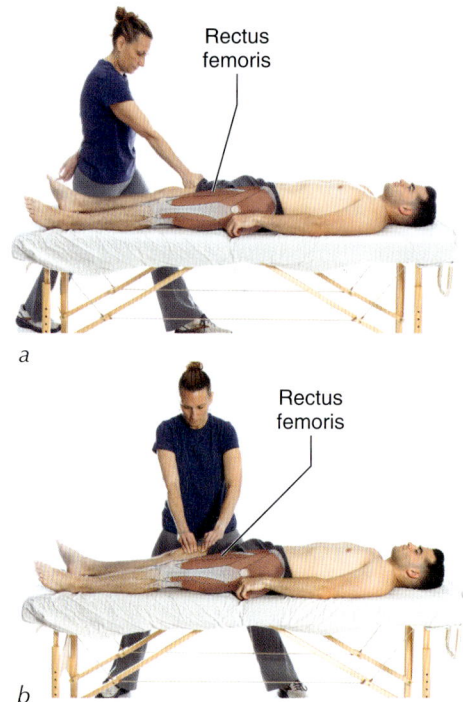

Figure 9.5 *(a)* Begin with glides on the rectus femoris. *(b)* The rectus femoris, once warmed, lends itself to lifting and shifting to release the fascia lata.

Medial Thigh

Treatment for the medial thigh can easily be done in a *figure-four position*, in which the patient is lying supine with the leg to be worked externally rotated at the hip and the knee in flexion (figure 9.6). The figure-four position places the muscles of the medial thigh facing up. If the patient does not have enough flexibility to rest the leg on the table, the foot can be crossed on the other leg and a bolster (or pillow or blanket) can be used under the bent knee to support the leg while it is being worked on. Alternately, the same techniques can be done with the patient in a side-lying position on the side being treated so that the medial aspect of the thigh is facing up.

Care needs to be taken with your body positioning. Although facing the patient allows you to read visual cues and maintain eye contact, use care in working toward the pelvic region, regardless of gender or sex. Facing away from the patient allows you to traction the muscles off the pubic and ischial bones; however, maintaining communication with your patient when your back is turned is of the utmost importance to continue to gauge pressure and to continue to check in with the patient for comfort. Also, to avoid being invasive, have the patient provide a manual barrier by putting their hand across the inguinal region. Doing so will keep you from crossing into an area that neither

Chapter 9 Hip, Thigh, and Knee

of you wants to invade with the treatment. It is acceptable to work this region without working all the way to the pubic bone attachments.

Following a warm-up with the spiral technique of the thigh, the medial aspect of the thigh can be treated with glides or with a traction compression. For glides, using the loose fist is preferred, especially if working distally to proximally. Glides can be done distally to proximally or proximally to distally along the medial aspect of the thigh, addressing some of the more medial aspect of the vastus medialis, which also attaches to the linea aspera, as well as the adductors. When working more laterally on the thigh, be sure to engage the fascial attachment between the adductor magnus and the semimembranosus. If glides are not effective or if the area is irritated, use a loose fist to traction the muscles off the pubic bone. Engage the muscles with a loose fist using compression that is less down into the tissue and more along the tissue toward the knee. Allow the tissue under your fist to release before disengaging and moving to another area on the medial thigh. Traction should not be used if there is any lubricant on the thigh, meaning it should ideally be done before any glides that use lubricant.

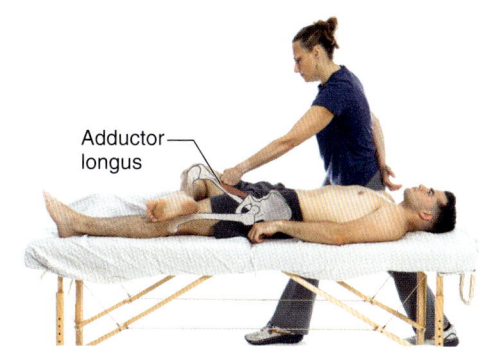

Figure 9.6 The patient is positioned with the foot resting just above the opposite knee. The therapist is using a loose fist engaged in the adductors.

To add to the technique, the patient can provide movement in the form of a pelvic tilt. Depending on the muscles of concern, the patient may feel the technique more with an anterior tilt (for the more posterior muscles) or a posterior tilt (for the more anterior muscles). All of these treatments are done more regionally rather than specific to the muscle.

Considerations for Medial Thigh Treatments

Keep in mind that the skin on the medial aspect of the thigh is sometimes very sensitive, and the fascia lata is typically a bit thinner (less dense) in this area. Be careful with glides. Traction techniques may be more appropriate to avoid irritating the skin. Alternatively, a small bit of low-drag lubricant (see chapter 3) may be used to allow for glides without distracting from fascial engagement.

Posterior Thigh

The posterior thigh can be treated in both the prone and supine positions, and both will be explained here. Whereas the prone position allows for easier access to the entire length of the hamstrings from the ischial tuberosity to the tibia and fibula, the supine position can be used to work the distal aspect of the hamstring group and incorporate active movement against gravity by the patient. In a treatment, it is possible to work both the proximal and distal hamstrings or to choose one based on the desired outcome. However, even if that session's treatment focuses on either the proximal or distal area, a comprehensive treatment plan addresses both areas, even if one does not seem to be the cause of the issue.

Like the rest of the thigh treatments, spiraling is used to warm the thigh. Spiraling is best done with the patient in the supine position, and it should be completed prior to turning the patient prone if that is the desired treatment. In the prone position, a great treatment for the proximal attachment of the hamstrings is compression at the ischial tuberosity (figure 9.7). Face the patient's feet, placing the proximal third of your ulna as a kind elbow against the ischial tuberosity. The compression against the ischial tuberosity can be held static, or you can gently rotate your forearm between pronation and supination to create some movement. Alternately, you can gently use a windshield-wiper motion, with alternating internal and external rotation of your shoulder providing the movement against the ischial tuberosity. Passively moving the patient's knee between flexion and extension can also be used as part of the treatment to the origin.

Cautions for the Massage Therapist

As the clinician, using your olecranon process is not advised because the ulnar nerve is exposed and easily irritated with too much pressure. Nothing concerns me more than when untrained clinicians claim they have already developed issues so they continue to use the point of their elbow and disregard their own safety, instead of taking the positive approach for their future.

Treatment of the muscle belly involves a series of glides, using any of your tools (forearm, loose fist, or heel of the hand) from distally to proximally. Glides over the lateral aspect of the thigh will treat both heads of the biceps femoris, whereas glides on the medial aspect will treat the semitendinosus (superficial) and the semimembranosus (deep). To further the treatment, move the knee passively into

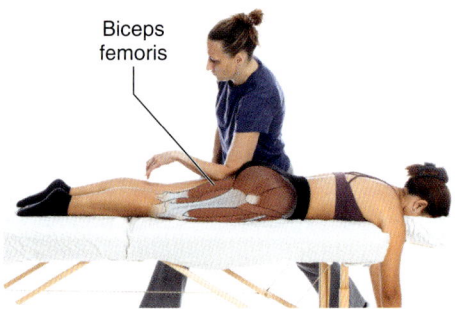

Figure 9.7 The therapist is in a lunge position, getting low enough to place the proximal third of the ulna against the ischial tuberosity. Pressure can be increased by lowering the lunge or using the body to lean back into the structure. More subtle pressure can be added with slow movement of the forearm.

flexion, and then glide distally to proximally with either passive or active extension of the knee. The movement should be slow, matching the speed of the glides. For the supine position, you are seated on the side of the table; the patient is positioned with their hip in flexion and their knee in flexion, resting on your shoulder (figure 9.8*b*). Place your outside hand on the patient's anterior thigh (if treating their right leg, it would be your left hand), bracing their leg. Using the inside forearm (if treating their right leg, it would be your right forearm), engage into the muscles and glide proximally to distally. In this treatment, have the patient slowly and actively extend their leg either during a static hold (pin and stretch) or a glide (figure 9.8). When you are ready, ask the patient to "kick to the ceiling." To emphasize the biceps femoris, position your forearm more laterally; to emphasize the semitendinosus and the semimembranosus, position your forearm more medially, working as much of the muscle as possible. The supine treatment is especially effective when working with more muscular and stronger patients.

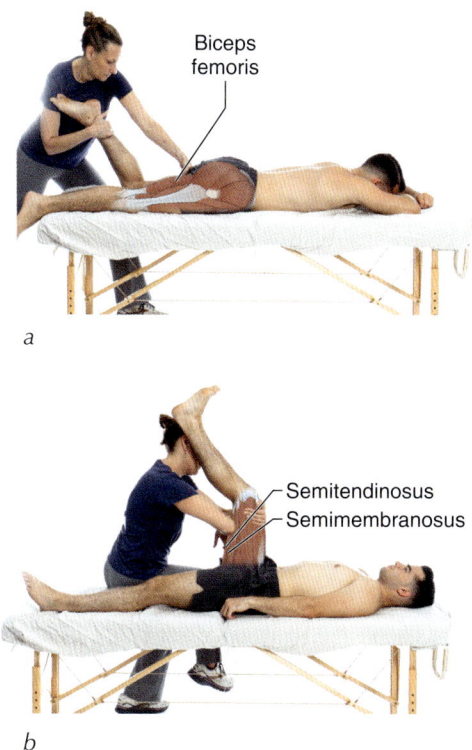

Figure 9.8 *(a)* The prone position where the emphasis can be more on the proximal portion of the muscle, while *(b)* the shows the pin and stretch with more patient engagement in the supine position.

POSTERIOR (GLUTEAL) REGION

The gluteal region is found posteriorly from the iliac crest, along the border of the sacrum to the ischial tuberosity and the greater trochanter. The area is covered by the very large gluteus maximus. Additionally, the thoracolumbar fascia superiorly becomes the gluteal fascia, which transitions to the posterior aspect of the fascia lata of the thigh. Transmission of forces up and down the kinetic chain can result in dysfunction in the gluteal area.

Muscles

Posteriorly, the gluteus maximus is superficial, covering all the other muscles, except for a slip of the gluteus medius found on the lateral side of the ilium. Treatment to all the deeper muscles including the piriformis, done in the prone position, relies on working through the gluteus maximus.

Gluteus Maximus

Origin
- Posterior one-fourth of the iliac crest
- Posterior surface of the sacrum
- Coccyx and the lumbar fascia

Insertion
- Bony attachment to the gluteal tuberosity on the femur
- Ridge on the lateral greater trochanter
- Fascial attachment into the iliotibial band of the fascia lata

Action
- Extension of the hip (acetabulofemoral joint)
- External rotation of the hip (acetabulofemoral joint)
- Upper fibers produce hip abduction (acetabulofemoral joint)
- Lower fibers produce hip adduction (acetabulofemoral joint); bilaterally produces posterior pelvic rotation

Innervation
- Inferior gluteal nerve

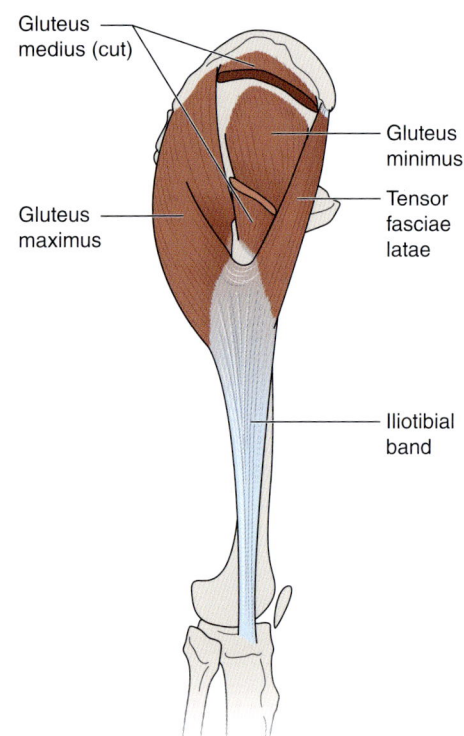

Figure 9.9 A lateral view of the gluteal muscles showing the arrangement of the gluteus minimus, gluteus medius, and gluteus maximus.

Chapter 9 Hip, Thigh, and Knee

Stressor Considerations

The gluteus maximus (figure 9.9) is responsible for forceful hip extension, such as when performing box jumps or squats or climbing stairs. The hamstring group, our other hip extensors, remains responsible for quiet hip extension, such as the extension used in walking on level ground. The gluteus maximus is a phasic muscle that can become inhibited secondary to the stresses put on it. For example, proper sitting posture involves sitting up straight on the ischial tuberosities (if you are sitting when you read this, I am guessing you readjusted your posture with the reminder… or at least I know I did while writing this!). If the pelvis is tucked under, like with a posterior pelvic tilt, the person ends up sitting on the gluteus maximus. The pressure from sitting on the gluteus maximus instead of the ischial tuberosity can lead to compression of the muscle, which will decrease blood flow to the area, leading to some of the negative effects of compressing a muscle (myofascial adhesions or myofascial trigger points). These negative effects can lead to inhibition of the muscle fibers, preventing the gluteus maximus from firing for more explosive movements. Treatment of the muscle, along with simple muscle reeducation exercises (I see you, bird dogs and fire hydrants!), can lead to optimal use of the gluteus maximus.

Deep Rotators of the Hip

The six external rotators of the hip are responsible for external rotation. I like to refer to these muscles as the *piriformis and the deep five* (gemellus superior, obturator internus, gemellus inferior, obturator externus, and quadratus femoris). They run from the ilium, ischium, and sacrum to the greater trochanter, and they are sometimes referred to as the *rotator cuff of the hip*. The piriformis, because of its relationship with the sciatic nerve, is often given the notoriety. These muscles are difficult to treat in isolation, so knowing the different muscle origins and insertions is great for an anatomy nerd but is not necessary to be a successful clinician. Therefore, the muscles are grouped together here as the piriformis and the deep five.

Piriformis

Origin
  Anterior sacrum
  Posterior portion of the ischium and the obturator foramen

Insertion
  Superior and posterior aspect of the greater trochanter

Action
  External rotation of the hip (acetabulofemoral joint)

Innervation
  First or second sacral nerve

Deep Five From Superior to Inferior by Origin

Gemellus superior
Obturator internus
Gemellus inferior
Obturator externus
Quadratus femoris

Stressor Considerations

Stressors of the piriformis and the deep five as a group come from externally rotating the hips, resulting in shortening of the muscles. The external rotation position can be secondary to creating a stable base for gait. Turning the feet out (externally rotating from the hip) and widening the base creates more stability for standing and walking. Examples include a baby learning how to walk, a pregnant woman adjusting her gait and center of gravity to accommodate the additional belly weight, or an individual with a neurological concern affecting his balance. Dancers also adopt a turnout with their feet, which is external rotation from the hip. Other individuals are also susceptible to these gait changes, or they may not have returned to their normal gait once the antalgic gait was adopted.

The piriformis, which gets top billing over the deep five, is often spoken about because of its relationship with the sciatic nerve. In typical anatomy, the sciatic nerve passes behind (deep to) the piriformis and can be compressed by a shortened and widened piriformis (its adaptation as a postural muscle). The shortening and widening decreases the allowable space for the sciatic nerve to pass. However, there are anatomical variations of the relationship in which the sciatic nerve passes over (superficial to) the piriformis, which adjusts its position. In another variation, one of the other branches of the sciatic nerve (the tibial or peroneal branch), which are normally maintained within the same sheath, passes over the piriformis (one superficial to and one deep to the piriformis). In yet another variation, one or both branches of the sciatic nerve could pass through (pierce) the piriformis (Travell and Simons 1983). With so many variations, effective piriformis treatment can vary from person to person. For example, direct compression that is too strong (greater than 8 on a scale of 1-10) would not be effective for someone who has one branch or both branches passing superiorly to the piriformis, because the nerve would be compressed when attempting to treat the muscle. Given these considerations, if the treatment clinicians know (compression) is not working, they should try something else in their tool kit.

Posterior (Gluteal) Region Treatment

With the patient positioned prone, compressions with a loose fist in the gluteal region are an ideal warm-up. It is very difficult to isolate muscles in this region; therefore, the treatment should work the entire region, from the iliac crest to the lateral edge of the sacrum to the greater trochanter. For the treatment, compressions can be concentrated to areas of particular tension. Additionally, you can use the proximal third of your forearm to cover larger areas of the muscle with the treatment. For this area, if you bend their knee, you can perform the treatment by concentrating your tool (loose fist or proximal third of the forearm) in one place and moving the muscle below your tool by internally and externally rotating the hip. This technique allows you to maintain a good, effective posture for treatment and still treat different areas of the muscle.

One specific treatment for the piriformis and the deep five is a pin and stretch. The piriformis is located between the greater trochanter and the lateral border of the sacrum, about at the middle third of the sacrum, and the rest of the rotators line up distally. Start by externally rotating the patient's hip to shorten the muscles. While using either a loose fist or the proximal third of the ulna, compress the tissues and hold, then slowly lengthen to stretch the muscles. This technique can be done down the length of the muscles. However, use caution and monitor for any increase in numbness and tingling that increases with the compression, as described earlier in the mention of stressor considerations.

Maintaining Appropriate Touch

As a clinician, I recommend not using an open hand on the gluteal area and instead relying on a loose fist or forearm. An open hand can simulate slapping or grabbing the buttocks, which might be offensive to some patients and is inappropriate.

Anterior Hip and Lateral Hip

The anterior hip and the lateral hip are grouped together here because of the common muscle treatments done in these areas. Anteriorly, clinicians can treat the rectus femoris (originating on the anterior inferior iliac spine [AIIS]), along with the sartorius (originating on the ASIS) and the tensor fasciae latae (originating on the ASIS). These three muscles create a superior triple attachment dubbed the Shiny (sartorius) Red (rectus femoris) Tomatoes (tensor fasciae latae). Whereas the rectus femoris and the sartorius are treated with the anterior thigh, the tensor fasciae latae can receive further treatment with the iliotibial band and the vastus lateralis when the client is in the side-lying position. The gluteus medius and the gluteus minimus can also be better accessed with the patient in a side-lying position compared with prone, although they will be affected somewhat when treating the gluteus maximus.

Because the muscles in the anterior and lateral hip area provide pull in different directions, the treatments will be slightly different, making palpation and muscle testing important for finding the key areas of treatment. As mentioned earlier, the sartorius and the tensor fasciae latae attach on the ASIS. Create a V sign with your index and third fingers and place them on the ASIS; the finger pointing medially represents the sartorius, and the finger pointing laterally represents the tensor fasciae latae. Directly between the two fingers, sitting deeper and attaching on the AIIS, is the rectus femoris. You will use this palpation trick to set up the triple attachment treatment described herein.

When the patient is in the side-lying position for the lateral hip treatment, you can use the iliac crest and the midline of the thigh (or the seam of their pants) to create the palpation navigation. Distal to the iliac crest and anterior to the midline of the lateral thigh to the ASIS, the tensor fasciae latae sits in its own little pocket. Distal to the iliac crest, posterior to the midline, and superior to the greater trochanter, the gluteus medius sits superficially with the gluteus minimus deep to it. Treating the gluteus minimus requires working through the gluteus medius.

Gluteus Medius

Origin
　Lateral surface of the ilium from just below the iliac crest to the anterior gluteal line

Insertion
　Posterior and middle surfaces of the greater trochanter of the femur

Action
　Abduction of the hip (acetabulofemoral joint)
　Anterior fibers produce internal rotation and flexion of the hip (acetabulofemoral joint)
　Posterior fibers produce external rotation and extension of the hip (acetabulofemoral joint)
　Lateral pelvic tilt

Innervation
　Superior gluteal nerve

Stressor Considerations

As pointed out with its actions, the gluteus medius as an abductor will also laterally tilt the pelvis. Think about a lateral pelvic tilt: When someone stands on the ground (closed-chain position) and abducts the hip, this essentially lifts one side of the pelvis superiorly, creating a lateral pelvic tilt. Therefore, if the person adopts any position with a lateral pelvic tilt, one side of the gluteus medius is automatically shortened and the contralateral side is lengthened. Weakness in the gluteus medius, whether secondary to the muscle being weak or inefficient in firing or as a response to fascial restrictions or trigger points, can lead to Trendelenburg gait, which occurs where there is a failure to maintain a level pelvis (lateral pelvic drop) during running or walking.

Gluteus Minimus

Origin
　Lateral surface of the ilium between the anterior and inferior gluteal lines

Insertion
　Anterior surface of the greater trochanter of the femur

Action
　Abduction of the hip (acetabulofemoral joint)
　Internal rotation of the hip (acetabulofemoral joint)
　Flexion of the hip (acetabulofemoral joint)
　Lateral pelvic tilt

Innervation
　Superior gluteal nerve

Stressor Considerations

The gluteus minimus is always completely covered by other muscles. Sometimes it is just deep to the gluteus medius; other times, it is deep to both the gluteus medius and gluteus maximus. In this situation, stressors to both muscles can transfer into the gluteus minimus. Therefore, treatment of the gluteus minimus is always through at least one other muscle layer.

Tensor Fasciae Latae

Origin
Anterior superior iliac spine

Anterior iliac crest

External surface of the ilium below the crest

Insertion
Into the iliotibial tract that ultimately inserts on Gerdy's tubercle on the anterolateral surface of the lateral tibial condyle

Function
Tenses the fascia lata

Action
Abduction of the hip (acetabulofemoral joint)

Internal rotation of the hip (acetabulofemoral joint)

Flexion of the hip (acetabulofemoral joint)

Lateral pelvic tilt

Innervation
Superior gluteal nerve

Stressor Considerations

The tensor fasciae latae are always depicted in anatomy texts as bright red muscle with white fascia coming from them. For those who have had the privilege of seeing cadaver anatomy (thank you to the wonderful donors who have taught me so much over the years), the tensor fasciae latae are actual muscle tissue embedded between layers of the fascia lata. They therefore appear white with distinct muscle fibers sandwiched between the fasciae. As the muscle fibers contract, they tense or pull the fascia lata, especially the overlap that forms the iliotibial band, in a superior direction. If the tensor fasciae latae muscle fibers are in a constant contracted state, they will pull the iliotibial band taut against the lateral femoral condyle and put pressure against the fat pad that sits at the distal end of the femur. This pulling up or shortening causes distal iliotibial band pain. If the band is pulled against the greater trochanter, this can lead to compression in the area of the greater trochanteric bursa as well as irritation, resulting in bursitis.

Sartorius

Origin
  Anterior superior iliac spine

Insertion
  Upper medial surface of the tibia below the medial condyle as part of the pes anserine group with the semitendinosus and the gracilis

Action
  Assists with flexion of the hip (acetabulofemoral joint)
  Abduction of the hip (acetabulofemoral joint)
  External rotation of the hip (acetabulofemoral joint)
  Flexion of the knee (tibiofemoral joint)

Innervation
  Femoral nerve

Stressor Considerations

The sartorius is the longest muscle in the body, sitting superficial to the anterior quadriceps group as it runs from lateral to medial across the thigh. This muscle has great range of motion, allowing for sitting with the legs crossed; however, the sartorius is not strong. The actions of the sartorius are only synergistic, assisting the prime movers. Rarely is the sartorius the cause of the problem; however, because it can be treated with all the other muscles, any problems can be easily addressed.

Anterior and Lateral Hip Treatment

Although the treatment described here is specific to the hip, these muscles also continue into the thigh, with some of them acting on the knee. Here, treatment of the anterior and lateral hip area is separated from the thigh treatments specific to the quadriceps and hamstrings, but these treatments may need to be used in conjunction with the thigh treatment to completely address the muscle. For example, only addressing the rectus femoris with the quadriceps group ignores its role in hip flexion, where it might be shortened as a result of prolonged sitting.

Anterior Treatment

The patient is positioned supine for the anterior treatment. Because all involved muscles, both anterior and lateral, cross onto the thigh or into the fascia lata, you can use the spiraling technique as a warm-up for this area. Even though the technique being done here addresses the superior attachment of the rectus femoris and the sartorius, it can be used with the treatment of the thigh as described earlier to create a complete treatment of the muscle. The tensor fasciae latae will be treated here and with the lateral treatment.

Using the palpation hints as described previously for the superior triple attachment, find the client's ASIS (figure 9.10). Line up your olecranon with the ASIS, and sink a kind elbow (more of the posterior border of the ulna) just below the ASIS. Sinking straight down will place the forearm on the superior aspect of the rectus femoris (figure 9.11). A gentle pronation and supination of your forearm can provide a gliding treatment in this stationary spot. To treat the sartorius, passively externally rotate the hip, allowing the sartorius to roll under the forearm, treating with the same gentle pronation and supination. To treat the tensor fasciae latae, internally rotate the hip, which will move the tensor fasciae latae under the forearm. The same gentle pronation and supination of the forearm is used here as well. Although this treatment is very short and simple, it is highly effective in this area.

Lateral Treatment

Place the patient in a side-lying position to work the lateral hip of the top leg (figure 9.12). The patient's head should be supported as comfortable, even if just with a pillow or their arm. Their bottom leg should be bent at the hip and knee, resting comfortably on the table. The top leg, the leg being worked, should be straight and ideally supported on a firm bolster or pillow (I like to use a foam roller). If you do not have a bolster, the patient's legs can be stacked, but their hips will drop into adduction and not be level in a relaxed, shortened position. If you are using an adjustable table, consider lowering the table to allow for good body mechanics to reach the area as their hips are stacked. If you are shorter or unable to drop the table, you can attempt to balance on a step stool, but be careful to maintain balance because your body mechanics will not allow for a good lunge position.

If you are addressing the tensor fasciae latae, iliotibial band, and lateral aspect of the vastus lateralis, start with spiraling and the anterior treatment before moving the patient to the side-lying position. Once the patient is in the side-lying position, use the iliac crest, ASIS, and midline of the lateral thigh to line up the muscle for

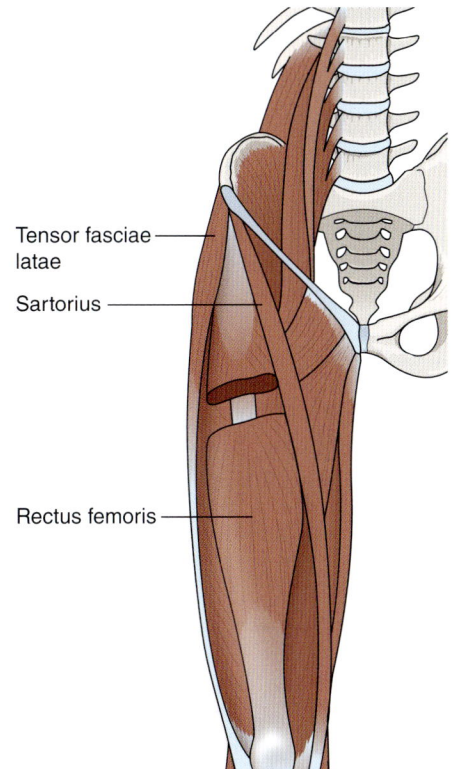

Figure 9.10 The three muscles—the tensor fasciae latae, sartorius, and rectus femoris—and their position in relation to the triple attachment technique at the ASIS and AIIS.

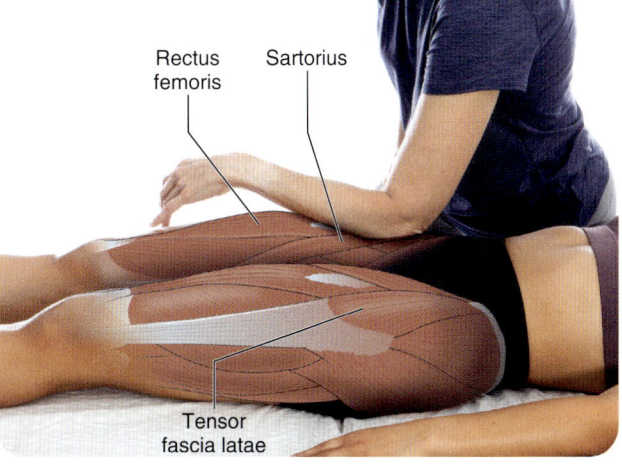

Figure 9.11 A kind elbow is used to sink into the space between the tensor fasciae latae and the sartorius where the rectus femoris sits. To change the muscle under the forearm, rotate the leg medially (tensor fasciae latae) or laterally (sartorius).

treatment (figure 9.12a). The tensor fasciae latae sits in an anterior pocket on the lateral iliac crest, which is where you place a kind elbow (proximal third of the ulna). As with the other treatments, you can enhance compression by using pronation and supination of the forearm or a gentle windshield-wiper motion. To add movement to the treatment, hold compression of the tensor fasciae latae and have the patient slowly move their top leg as if they were pedaling a bicycle about five times. Typically, the patient has some difficulty the first two times they move the leg, but the muscle releases and they can move freely by the third or fourth time.

To address the gluteus medius and the gluteus minimus, you can start with either spiraling and the anterior treatment or use this treatment in conjunction with the posterior gluteal treatment. If you are not doing either of those treatments, make sure to

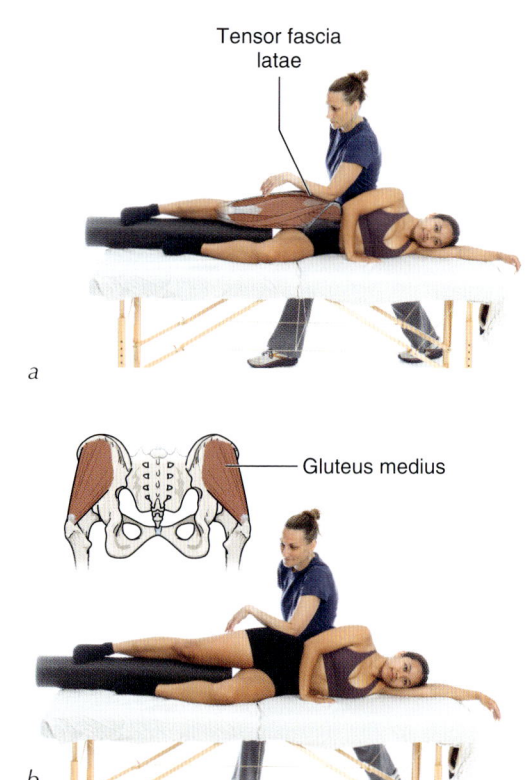

Figure 9.12 (a) Treatment for the tensor fasciae latae in the anterior aspect of the lateral ilium; (b) treatment for the gluteus medius (and gluteus minimus, which is deep to the gluteus medius), posterior to the midline of the lateral thigh.

do some gentle compressions with a loose fist to warm the area before beginning. This treatment is done on the lateral aspect of the external ilium, from the iliac crest to the greater trochanter, posterior to the midline of the lateral thigh (figure 9.12b). As with the tensor fasciae latae, use a kind elbow for compression. Pronation and supination of your forearm or application of a gentle windshield-wiper motion can enhance the treatment. If movement of the hip is desired, internal and external rotation of the hip is favored over flexion (as with the bicycle move just described).

Treatment for the lateral thigh, which should be done after warming the anterior thigh and releasing the tensor fasciae latae, includes glides from just superior to the lateral femoral condyle to the greater trochanter, making sure not to push too hard around the fat pad near the femoral condyle. For the iliotibial band, the best technique involves shifting the edge of the band to loosen the distal aspect. To achieve this, place your two thumbs at the distinct distal edge of the band (to differentiate from the biceps femoris, have the patient actively bend their knee; the tendon of the biceps femoris will have increased tension, whereas the iliotibial band will not). With the braced thumbs on the lateral edge of the band, push anteriorly with the thumbs (not down into the tissue, but across the edge) while bracing with the rest of

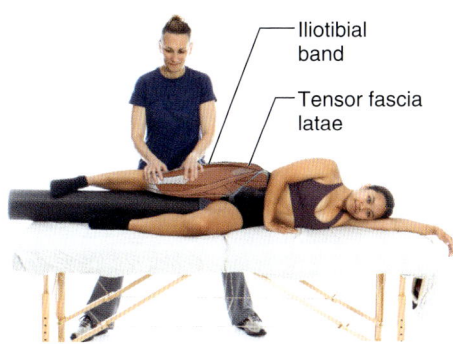

Figure 9.13 With braced thumbs, gently traction along the lateral aspect of the iliotibial band trying to mobilize it within the fascia latae.

the fingers as though you were bending a twig (not breaking or snapping the edges) (figure 9.13). Hold this position until the fascia softens, and then continue distally to proximally until the sharp edge of the band diminishes, anywhere from a third to two-thirds of the way superior on the lateral thigh.

WHY DOES THE CLINICIAN CARE?

From knee and hip surgeries to acute hamstring strains to overuse injuries such as iliotibial band syndrome, the muscles of the hip and thigh, surrounded by the fascia lata, respond well to massage treatments. The large surface areas benefit from more broad techniques (as opposed to focused techniques of the foot or hand) and from techniques such as the pin and stretch, which allow for adding dynamic movement. Whether the clinician is working with an athlete or someone who is on their feet all day for work (e.g., an occupational athlete), massage to the hip and thighs can help relieve muscle tension and soreness.

10

Lower Leg and Foot

For manual therapy, it is helpful to look at the lower leg and foot from the ground up, which is more of a functional and sport perspective, rather than from the knee down, which is more of an anatomical perspective. The foot features an arch structure that creates a three-legged stool with points at the calcaneus, first metatarsal head, and fifth metatarsal head, while also uniquely having the ability to absorb and transfer forces. The lower leg has an intricate structure of muscle compartments and fascia to allow for movements of the ankle, the foot, and even the knee.

Joint Structure

The lower leg consists of joints between the tibia and the fibula, which are nonmoving, and the ankle joint, which is a combination of two joints. The foot features a structure similar to the hand, in which the tarsal bones form gliding joints with each other and the metatarsal bones. The phalanges of the foot create a joint structure similar to the fingers of the hand.

Lower Leg

The tibia and fibula have proximal and distal gliding joints that do not allow for any actions. Especially proximally, there is little movement of the head of the fibula as it rests against the lateral tibial condyle. With two bones in the lower leg, there is increased surface area for muscle attachments. These muscles are divided into four distinct compartments:

1. The *anterior compartment* made up of the tibialis anterior, the extensor hallucis longus, the extensor digitorum longus, and the peroneus tertius
2. The *lateral compartment* made up of the peroneus longus and the peroneus brevis
3. The *superficial posterior compartment* made up of the gastrocnemius, the soleus, and the plantaris
4. The *deep posterior compartment* made up of the posterior tibialis, the flexor hallucis longus, the flexor digitorum longus, and the popliteus

The *interosseus membrane* is a thick, supportive connective tissue between the tibia and fibula (figure 10.1). Based on the arrangement of the fibers, the interosseus membrane provides a bit of downward pull, helping to keep the fibula in place against the tibia. The interosseus membrane creates an area for muscle attachment as well as a divider between the anterior compartment and the deep posterior compartment of the lower leg. The membrane also serves to increase the surface area for muscle attachments compared to if there were one bone in the lower leg, and it better allows for the transfer of forces.

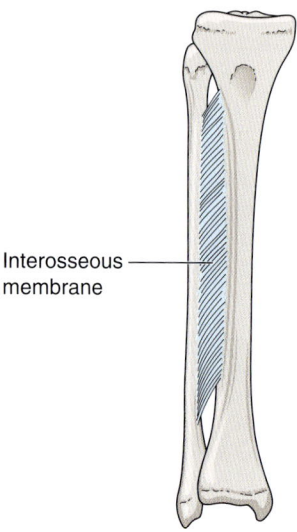

Figure 10.1 The interosseus (inter = between; osseus = bone) membrane increases the surface area for muscle attachment in the low leg, helps to distribute forces, and serves to divide the anterior and deep posterior compartments.

Ankle

The ankle is a series of two joints: the talocrural joint and the subtalar joint. The *talocrural joint* is the articulation between the talus, tibia, and fibula, where the talus moves between the two bones of the lower leg. The talocrural joint is a hinge joint, allowing for plantar flexion and dorsiflexion. The *subtalar joint* is the articulation between the inferior aspect of the talus on the calcaneus. Like the rest of the intertarsal joints, the subtalar joint is a gliding joint; however, the subtalar joint produces inversion and eversion of the ankle, whereas the rest of the intertarsal joints glide on one another without producing a distinct action.

Because multiple tarsal bones plus the tibia and fibula are involved in the ankle, there are many ligaments. The ligaments discussed here are those most likely to be involved in an ankle sprain. The most common mechanism for an ankle sprain is inversion of the calcaneus, meaning the most common ligaments sprained are the three on the lateral side: the anterior talofibular ligament, the posterior talofibular ligament, and the calcaneofibular ligament. An eversion mechanism would result in injury to the ligament on the medial side of the ankle, the more complex deltoid ligament. In a syndesmosis sprain (also termed a *high ankle sprain*), the mechanism of injury is extreme dorsiflexion with eversion, resulting in a sprain of the tibiofibular ligaments and even the interosseus membrane.

Foot

Regions of the foot include the rearfoot, the midfoot, and the forefoot. The foot includes all 7 tarsal bones as well as the 5 metatarsal bones and the 14 phalanx bones that make up the 5 phalanges. As with the hand, the foot has three bones each in the four lesser toes (a proximal phalange, a middle phalange, and a distal phalange) and two phalanges in the first toe or *hallux* (a proximal phalange and a distal phalange).

INTERTARSAL JOINTS
The joints in the foot, outside of the subtalar joint, are all gliding joints that do not produce a distinct action but do glide on one another. The series of joints includes the intertarsal joints (between two tarsal bones) and the tarsometatarsal joints (between the distal row of tarsal bones and the five metatarsal bones). These bones are held together in a structure supported by ligaments and fascia as well as the intrinsic muscles of the foot.

PHALANGEAL JOINTS
The foot and the hand look very similar in terms of structure of the metatarsophalangeal joints and interphalangeal joints. The *metatarsophalangeal joints* are condyloid or ellipsoidal, producing the actions of flexion and extension as well as abduction, adduction, and circumduction. There is no saddle joint in the foot as there is in the hand. The *interphalangeal joints* are hinge joints producing only flexion and extension, with two joints in each of the four lesser toes and one joint in the hallux.

ARCHES
The foot has three arches: a medial arch, a lateral longitudinal arch, and a transverse arch, which includes the metatarsal arch anteriorly. These arches form a three-dimensional structure (similar to a three-legged stool on which people can stand and propel themselves during movement), along with connective tissue structures, muscle tendons, ligaments, and the plantar fascia. The arches of the foot provide flexibility and shock absorption as well propulsion during both walking and running. The bones, tendons, and ligaments of the foot working together are responsible for the combination of absorbing and redistributing forces through the flexibility of the structures with the ability to form a rigid lever for propulsion. The arches also allow humans to adapt to different surfaces; for example, think about differences in walking barefoot on sand, grass, and a hard-surface floor. The foot adapts to the surface while still allowing for propulsion.

The keystone of the medial longitudinal arch is the navicular bone, which holds up and supports the rest of the bony structures. Supporting the arch passively is the plantar calcaneonavicular ligament (or spring ligament), with the posterior tibialis tendon providing dynamic stability. If the foot is too supple, it absorbs too much force into the soft tissues. If the foot is too rigid, force is not absorbed adequately, which can lead to dysfunction in the bones. During gait, the concerted movement of the bones in the arch and soft tissue allows people to efficiently absorb forces and then use those forces to propel themselves forward in motion. The body's inability to adequately absorb and redistribute these forces can lead to injury over time. For manual therapy, it is important for the clinician to provide appropriate treatments to the muscles, allowing them to work correctly in the gait cycle to adequately absorb and redistribute forces.

PLANTAR FASCIA

The plantar fascia is a large, multilayered connective tissue structure. It originates near the calcaneal tubercle, the insertion of the Achilles tendon, and runs into the metatarsals. The plantar fascia provides more supple support for the plantar surface of the foot, acting as a shock absorber in weight-bearing activity. Of concern with treating the plantar fascia is the presence of inflammation as a cause of pain. Manual therapy treatments that increase inflammation may cause more pain in the area and continue the cycle of pain and inflammation. As seen with some other areas of treatment, working the muscles around the area can be helpful in treating the plantar fascia without exacerbating inflammation.

LIGAMENTS

The foot has numerous ligaments as part of the various joints. It is not unusual for an athlete to receive a foot sprain diagnosis without indication of which ligament is involved. The plantar calcaneonavicular ligament, which connects the calcaneus with the navicular bone, is a major passive support of the medial longitudinal arch. Acute injury to this ligament can lead to dysfunction in the arch. From another perspective, someone lacking a medial longitudinal arch (i.e., flatfoot or *pes planus*) may develop laxity in the ligament over time. Regardless of the ligaments injured in the foot, strengthening and treating the muscles will assist in returning to a normal and pain-free gait.

MUSCLES OF THE LOWER LEG

As mentioned earlier, the muscles of the lower leg are divided into four compartments: anterior, lateral, superficial posterior, and deep posterior. Included in the lower leg are extrinsic muscles that produce flexion and extension of the toes, as well as the four major movements at the ankle: plantar flexion, dorsiflexion, inversion, and eversion. The intrinsic muscles of the plantar surface of the foot can also be divided into layers and will be discussed here in general. Proprioception is also a key function of the muscles of the lower leg.

Anterior Compartment

The anterior compartment of the lower leg includes the muscles that produce dorsiflexion and are located lateral to the tibia and medial to the fibula. Treatment will focus on this area. All of the muscles pass anteriorly to the malleoli, directing their line of pull in the sagittal plane to produce dorsiflexion. The medial muscles also produce inversion, whereas the lateral muscles produce eversion.

The tibialis anterior is the most superficial of the muscles and is the main muscle of dorsiflexion. Joining the tibialis anterior are the extensor digitorum longus, the extensor hallucis longus (the extrinsic extensors of the phalanges), and the peroneus tertius (figure 10.2). These muscles are typically phasic in nature and weaker than the larger, stronger plantar flexors.

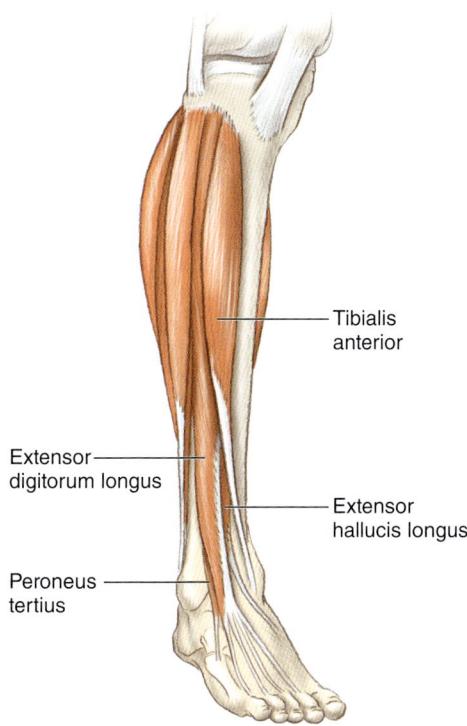

Figure 10.2 Muscles of the anterior compartment sit between the lateral aspect of the tibia and the medial aspect of the fibula. They cross anterior to the malleoli.

Tibialis Anterior

Origin
Upper two-thirds of the lateral portion of the tibia

Insertion
Inner surface of the medial cuneiform and the base of the first metatarsal

Action
Dorsiflexion of the ankle (talocrural joint)
Inversion of the foot (subtalar joint)

Innervation
Deep peroneal nerve

Stressor Considerations

As the main muscle of dorsiflexion, the tibialis anterior is involved in controlling eccentric plantar flexion. Think about walking downhill: The ankle needs to plantar flex to meet the ground. The tibialis anterior helps to control the ankle and slow down the plantar flexion, preventing the foot from slapping the ground. Weakness in the tibialis anterior is associated with gait abnormalities such as foot drop or foot slap (including injuries to the deep peroneal nerve). Because this small muscle is fighting the stronger muscles of plantar flexion, it is often a victim of this muscle imbalance.

Extensor Digitorum Longus

Origin
Lateral condyle of the tibia
Head of the fibula
Upper anterior surface of the fibula

Insertion
Splits into four tendons that insert into the head of the middle and distal phalanges of the four lesser toes

Action
Extension of the four lesser toes at the metatarsophalangeal, proximal interphalangeal, and distal interphalangeal joints
Assists with dorsiflexion of the ankle (talocrural joint) and eversion of the foot (subtalar joint)

Innervation
Deep peroneal nerve

Stressor Considerations

The extensor digitorum longus is typically eccentrically strained. Much of how people use the foot involves gripping with the muscles on the plantar surface, producing flexion of the toes. As a result, muscles such as the extensor digitorum longus and the extensor digitorum brevis on the dorsal surface of the foot tend to be lengthened.

Extensor Hallucis Longus

Origin
   Middle two-thirds of the medial surface of the anterior fibula

Insertion
   Base of the distal phalanx of the hallux (first or great toe)

Action
   Extension of the hallux at the metatarsophalangeal and interphalangeal joints
   Assists with dorsiflexion of the ankle (talocrural joint) and inversion of the foot (subtalar joint)

Innervation
   Deep peroneal nerve

Stressor Considerations

Unlike the rest of the muscles in the anterior compartment, the tendon for the extensor hallucis longus may be stressed with the normal gait cycle. The toe-off gait position requires extension of the hallux at the first metatarsal phalangeal joint. Injuries such as a sprain of the first metatarsal phalangeal joint (*turf toe*) can lead to stress on the muscle belly, located in the lower leg.

Peroneus Tertius

Origin
   Distal third of the anterior fibula

Insertion
   Superior aspect of the base of the fifth metatarsal

Action
   Dorsiflexion of the ankle (talocrural joint)
   Eversion of the foot (subtalar joint)

Innervation
   Deep peroneal nerve

Stressor Considerations

The peroneus tertius, the third peroneal muscle, is absent in a percentage of the population. Although the peroneus tertius may not be a muscle of injury concern, it is treated with the rest of the muscles in its compartment.

Anterior Compartment of the Lower Leg Treatment

The entire anterior compartment can be treated as a unit, working through the superficial anterior tibialis to get to the bellies of the other muscles. For this manual therapy treatment, place the patient supine. You will work from the foot of the table. For a good warming technique, perform myofascial glides distally to proximally, laterally to the tibia, and medially to the fibula. You can do these glides using the heel of your hand or a loose fist, with your wrist straight and your forearm positioned between pronation and supination. You can also perform these glides with movement, starting with the patient's ankle in dorsiflexion (shortened) and slowly gliding proximally while bringing the ankle into plantar flexion (lengthening). Similar glides can be done using a combination of dorsiflexion to plantar flexion with inversion and eversion.

A second technique can be done from the side of the table, facing the lower leg. You can use braced thumbs (right and left thumbs supporting each other) to traction the muscles off the tibia and interosseus membrane (figure 10.3). This action helps to release the muscles from the fascial attachments.

With the patient in the same supine position, you can perform glides across the retinaculum, which serves to keep the tendons in place, allowing them to keep the direct line of pull for muscle efficiency. Because the retinacula are extensions of the deep fascia covering the lower leg, restrictions can prevent the effective eccentric movement of the muscles during plantar flexion.

Cautions for the Anterior Compartment

Avoid performing glides or compression directly on the anterior surface of the tibia. Think about how uncomfortable it is when you bang your shin; do not bang the patient's shin.

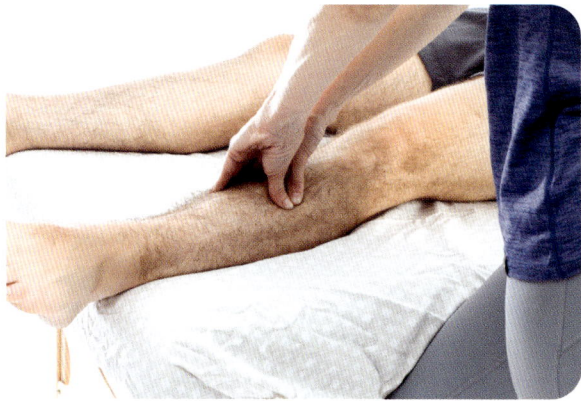

Figure 10.3 Braced thumbs are used to sink into the anterior compartment, providing traction of the muscle from the tibia and interosseus membrane using slow engagement in the tissue. The technique is performed along the entire length of the lower leg.

Lateral Compartment

The lateral compartment is located along the fibula (figure 10.4). Place one finger on the head of the fibula and one on the lateral malleolus; notice that the muscles run between the two spots. The tendons then cross behind the lateral malleolus, which influences the line of pull to produce plantar flexion and eversion. Because the two muscle bellies overlap in the central portion of the fibula, treatment is difficult to isolate.

The peroneal muscles are often stressed with a lateral ankle sprain when the foot is inverted. In addition to their actions, they function as being highly proprioceptive. These two bits of information emphasize the importance of treating any potential areas of concern in the muscles, such as after an ankle sprain or in chronic ankle instability.

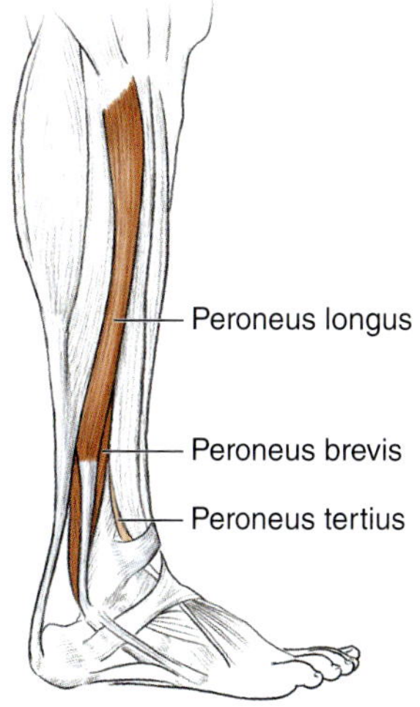

Figure 10.4 The two muscles of the lateral compartment are the peroneus longus and the peroneus brevis. The peroneus tertius is in the anterior compartment.

Peroneus Longus

Origin
Upper two-thirds of the lateral aspect of the fibula

Insertion
Plantar surface of the medial cuneiform and the first metatarsal

Action
Plantar flexion of the ankle (talocrural joint); the muscle is weak in plantar flexion but highly proprioceptive

Eversion of the foot (subtalar joint)

Innervation
Superficial peroneal nerve

Stressor Considerations

In addition to ankle injury as mentioned earlier, the peroneus longus becomes part of the supporting structure of the arches in the foot. When the peroneus longus and posterior tibialis work together, they act as a sling to create a balance in the foot between inversion and eversion of the ankle, especially when balancing on one leg. The ability of these muscles to work together as stabilizers is a consideration not only of rehabilitation but also of manual therapy treatments.

Peroneus Brevis

Origin
Middle to lower two-thirds of the lateral surface of the fibula

Insertion
Tuberosity of the base of the fifth metatarsal

Action
Plantar flexion of the ankle (talocrural joint)
Eversion (subtalar joint)

Innervation
Superficial peroneal nerve

Stressor Considerations

The insertion at the base of the fifth metatarsal means the muscle may be stressed with a Jones fracture, which may require surgery, as well as with an ankle sprain. Otherwise, the stressors for the peroneus longus and the peroneus brevis are similar.

Lateral Compartment of the Lower Leg Treatment

Have the patient lie on the side not being treated, allowing the lateral aspect of the lower leg being treated to be facing toward you.

The patient's leg can be supported with a bolster under the medial side or the leg can rest on the table. If you plan to add movement and the patient is not bolstered, position the foot to allow for a full range of motion between eversion and inversion.

Treatment to the lateral compartment includes myofascial glides running from the lateral malleolus to just distal to the head of the fibula (figure 10.5). You can use the heel of your hand or a loose fist (the proximal phalanges work best because they allow for a neutral wrist). To add movement, start with passively placing the foot in eversion (shortening the muscle) and slowly bringing it passively into inversion with one hand while gliding distally to proximally with the other. As with the anterior compartment, the retinacula supporting the peroneal muscles may become stuck. Glides around (not over) the malleolus can be used to relieve the restrictions.

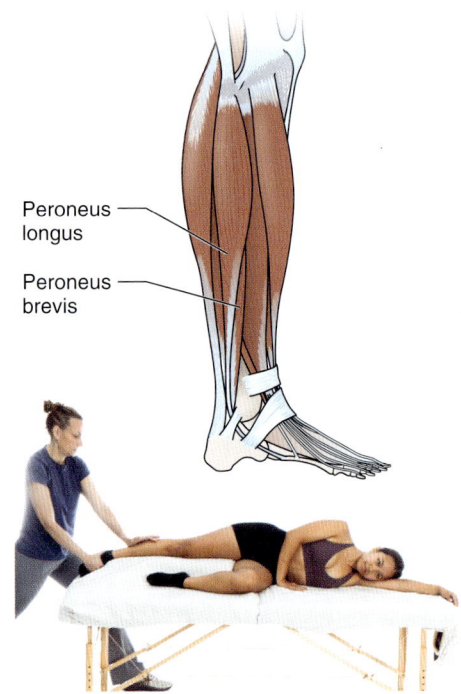

Figure 10.5 Glides are performed using the heel of the hand from distal to proximal. As the therapist's hand glides from just above the lateral malleolus to the fibular head, the foot is moved from eversion to inversion.

Cautions Around the Head of the Fibula

Because the peroneal nerve is superficial as it wraps around the head of the fibula, treatment should stop distal to the head of the fibula. Pressure directly over the head of the fibula should be avoided. Instruct the patient to speak up if any part of the treatment elicits the feeling of numbness and tingling.

Superficial Posterior Compartment

The superficial posterior compartment consists of the gastrocnemius and soleus along with the tendon from the plantaris muscle, which runs between the two muscle bellies (figure 10.6). The gastrocnemius, which has two heads, and the soleus, which has one, come together into the common Achilles tendon, with the plantaris inserting just medial on the calcaneus. From a palpation standpoint, the gastrocnemius is the most superficial, with two heads coming from the posterior aspect of the femur. Palpation of the soleus can be done just lateral to the gastrocnemius bellies and, depending on the client's anatomy, may appear inferior as well under the fascial layer.

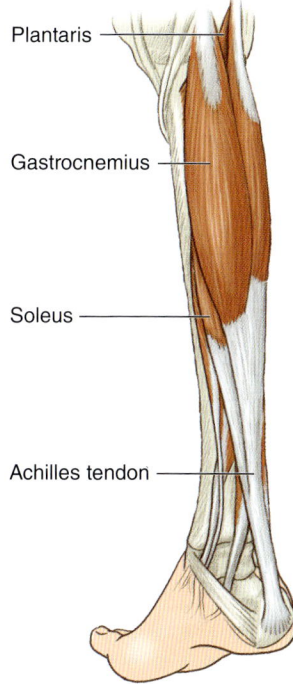

Figure 10.6 The muscles of the superficial posterior compartment consist of the gastrocnemius, soleus, and plantaris. The gastrocnemius has two heads and crosses the knee as well as the ankle. The soleus only crosses the ankle, making it the stronger plantarflexor. The belly of the plantaris is in the popliteal space, and the tendon runs between gastrocnemius and soleus.

All three muscles in the superficial posterior compartment perform plantar flexion, with action only in the sagittal plane. Because the soleus does not cross the knee, it is the strongest of the muscles that plantar flex the ankle. The plantaris is the smallest and does not contribute much strength to the action. All of these muscles are postural, responding to stress by shortening.

Gastrocnemius

Origin
Medial head originates on the posterior surface of the medial femoral condyle

Lateral head originates on the posterior surface of the lateral femoral condyle

Insertion
The two heads join to form the Achilles tendon, eventually inserting on the posterior surface of the calcaneus

Action
Plantar flexion of the ankle (talocrural joint)

Flexion of the knee (tibiofemoral joint)

Innervation
Tibial nerve

Stressor Considerations
Any position that puts the ankle into continuous plantar flexion can stress the gastrocnemius. Examples of stressors include wearing shoes with a high heel, activity done on the toes, or even running on sand (or any soft surface that dissipates force). In addition, the relaxed or resting position of the leg is in plantar flexion, including during sleep. Cramps in the gastrocnemius are not uncommon, especially if the person is dehydrated or has an electrolyte deficiency. Effective treatment can be dependent on any of the stressors causing dysfunction in the muscle.

Soleus

Origin
Posterior surface of the proximal fibula

Proximal two-thirds of the posterior surface of tibia (distal to the soleal or popliteal line of the tibia)

Insertion
Joins the gastrocnemius to become part of the Achilles tendon, eventually inserting into the posterior surface of the calcaneus

Action
Plantar flexion of the ankle (talocrural joint)

Innervation
Tibial nerve

Stressor Considerations

The soleus is the workhorse of the plantar flexor group. It is the strongest muscle but is often overlooked because the gastrocnemius is more popular. To isolate the soleus for stretching, performing calf stretches with a bend in the knee (knee flexion) will remove the gastrocnemius and the plantaris from the stretch, because both muscles cross the knee and are activated with knee flexion.

Plantaris

Origin
Lower portion of the posterior aspect of the lateral femoral condyle (distal to the gastrocnemius)

Insertion
Posterior surface of the calcaneus medial to the Achilles tendon

Action
Plantar flexion of the ankle (talocrural joint)

Weak knee flexion (tibiofemoral joint)

Innervation
Tibial nerve

Stressor Considerations

The plantaris is a very weak muscle. Injury to the plantaris, including rupture, is often overlooked and thus may not be treated or repaired.

Superficial Posterior Compartment of the Lower Leg Treatment

The patient should be placed comfortably in the prone position. The foot can hang off the table, allowing for good movement between plantar flexion and dorsiflexion, or a bolster can be placed under the lower leg if range of motion can be achieved. Treatment of the superficial posterior compartment starts with warming techniques. You can use compression and petrissage prior to gentle myofascial glides (on the pressure scale from 1 to 10, use 4 or 5) to warm the area. Specific to the gastrocnemius, the glides should be performed distally to proximally from just proximal to the Achilles tendon to just below the popliteal space (figure 10.7). If you are treating the medial head of the gastrocnemius, work the glides medially toward the posterior aspect of the medial femoral condyle. When you are treating the lateral head of the gastrocnemius, work the glides laterally toward the posterior aspect of the lateral femoral condyle. Add movement from plantar flexion into dorsiflexion while gliding with the same parameters.

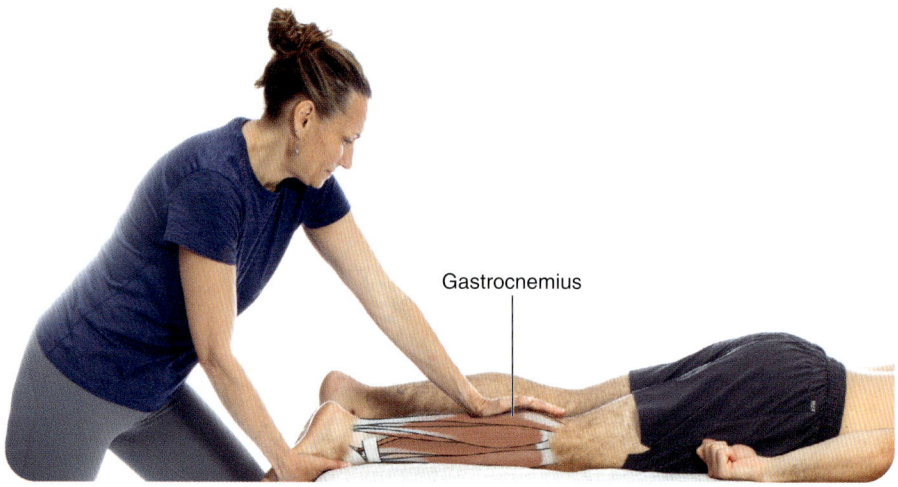

Figure 10.7 Treatment to the gastrocnemius includes glides to the muscle belly. The therapist is positioned at the end of the table with the patient's foot hanging off. The other hand can be used to bring the foot from plantar flexion into dorsiflexion.

Cautions Around the Popliteal Space

Avoid working directly in the popliteal space, because the blood vessels and nerves are superficial. Instead, work laterally toward the proximal attachments of each head of the gastrocnemius at the posterior aspect of the femoral condyle.

Once the gastrocnemius is warmed through, treatment to the deeper muscles can occur. The tendon of the plantaris will be worked with the gastrocnemius, and the origin can be worked with the lateral head of the gastrocnemius. To treat the soleus, it is possible to work through the gastrocnemius but also to work the medial and lateral aspects where the muscle is accessible. For this treatment, flexion of the knee can provide a better angle for you (figure 10.8). Using your fingertips, perform slow glides distally to proximally along the medial and lateral aspects of the muscle. If motion is desired, it is easier to have the patient perform active movement from plantar flexion to dorsiflexion than trying passive motion (remember to isolate the soleus, and maintain flexion in the knee).

Finally, you can use gentle pressure to mobilize the Achilles tendon (figure 10.9). Once the muscles are released, gently move the tendon medially and laterally using minimal pressure.

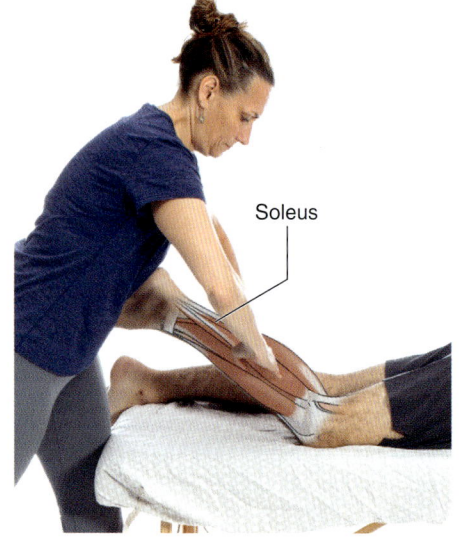

Figure 10.8 The therapist uses the fingertips to perform slow, sustained glides on the lateral and medial edges of the soleus, just deep to the gastrocnemius. Remember to keep the knee bent both for ease of the treatment for the clinician and for better access to soleus.

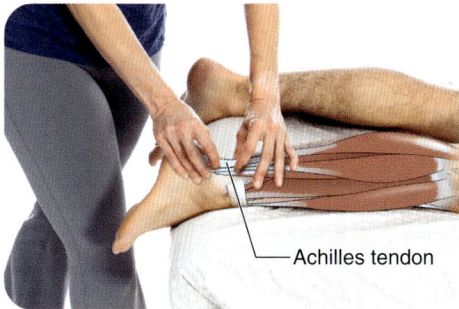

Figure 10.9 Gentle mobilization to the Achilles tendon is performed. Make sure to grasp the tendon and do not work deep onto the bursa.

Cautions Around the Achilles Tendon

Avoid working too deep, because there are bursae deep to the Achilles tendon that should not be squeezed. Also, some people do not like to have this work done to the Achilles, so always be mindful of patient preferences.

Deep Posterior Compartment

The deep posterior compartment sits posteriorly between the tibia and fibula and can be palpated along the medioposterior edge of the tibia (figure 10.10). Because of how deep the muscles sit, treatment cannot access the entirety of the muscle bellies. However, as in other areas, clinicians can work with the more superficial soft tissue structures and as much of these muscles as they can access. The muscle tendons pass behind the medial malleolus with the tibial artery, vein, and nerve in the following order: posterior tibialis, flexor digitorum longus, tibial artery, tibial vein, tibial nerve, and flexor hallucis longus. (To remember the order, try this mnemonic: Tom, Dick, and A Very Nervous Harry.)

The muscles of the deep posterior compartment all traverse behind the medial malleolus. The muscles produce inversion as well as weak plantar flexion. In addition,

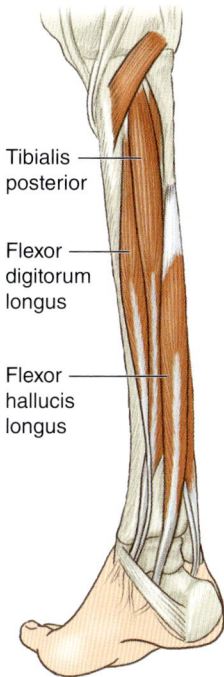

Figure 10.10 The deep posterior compartment sits deep to the superficial posterior compartment; however, the easiest way to access the muscles for treatment is medial to the tibia.

the flexor digitorum longus flexes the lesser toes, and the flexor hallucis longus flexes the hallux.

Posterior Tibialis

Origin
Posterior surface of the upper half of the interosseus membrane
Adjacent surfaces of the tibia and fibula

Insertion
Inferior surfaces of the navicular, cuneiform, and cuboid bones, as well as the bases of the second, third, and fourth metatarsals

Action
Plantar flexion of the ankle (talocrural joint)
Inversion of the foot (subtalar joint)

Innervation
Tibial nerve

Stressor Considerations

The posterior tibialis has a large connective tissue attachment to the interosseus membrane and is located in the area of pain for people diagnosed with medial tibial stress syndrome (sometimes incorrectly termed *shin splints*). The posterior tibialis also works with the peroneus longus as a sling, creating balance to the plantar surface of the foot by supporting the arches. *Pes planus*, where the medial longitudinal arch is dropped, is often associated with medial tibial stress syndrome. In looking at these connections, the question becomes this: Is the dysfunction in the posterior tibialis a cause of medial shin pain or a result? Either way, treatment to release the muscle may assist in any fascial restrictions. However, use caution if a stress fracture is diagnosed or suspected in the area.

Flexor Digitorum Longus

Origin
Middle third of the posterior surface of the tibia

Insertion
Splits into four tendons that insert on the base of the distal phalanx of each of the lesser four toes

Action
Flexion of the four lesser toes at the metatarsophalangeal, proximal interphalangeal, and distal interphalangeal joints
Weak in plantar flexion of the ankle (talocrural joint) and inversion of the foot (subtalar joint)

Innervation
Tibial nerve

Chapter 10 Lower Leg and Foot

Stressor Considerations

The flexor digitorum longus is the extrinsic muscle responsible for flexion of the toes. It shares an unusual relationship with the lumbrical muscles that attach to the tendons on the plantar surface of the foot. In addition, because the tendon crosses behind the medial malleolus, the angle of pull for the muscle is inefficient. Therefore, the quadratus plantae, originating on the calcaneus, inserts into the flexor digitorum tendon and serves to realign the pull of the flexor digitorum longus. Considering the additional structures aligning with the muscle, full treatment of the flexor digitorum longus should include treatment to the deep posterior compartment and the plantar surface of the foot.

Flexor Hallucis Longus

Origin
  Middle two-thirds of the posterior surface of the fibula

Insertion
  Base of the plantar surface of the distal phalanx of the hallux (first or great toe)

Action
  Flexion of the metatarsophalangeal and interphalangeal joints of the hallux
  Weak plantar flexion of the ankle (talocrural joint) and inversion of the foot (subtalar joint)

Innervation
  Tibial nerve

Stressor Considerations

As mentioned for the extensor hallucis longus, the toe-off motion is an important part of gait. Therefore, the flexor hallucis longus works as an antagonist to the extension produced by the extensor hallucis longus.

Deep Posterior Compartment of the Lower Leg Treatment

Treatment of the deep posterior compartment should follow a thorough warm-up of the superficial musculature in the superficial posterior compartment. Although treatment of the entire superficial posterior compartment may not be necessary, the clinician should provide a sufficient warm-up to ensure the deep posterior compartment is ready for the treatment.

Positioning for the deep posterior treatment is best done with the patient lying on the affected side, so the medial aspect of the tibia is facing up (figure 10.11). The leg can rest comfortably on the table, either with the leg straight (with the top leg knee bent, crossed over comfortably, and bolstered) or with the opposite leg straight (with the top leg bolstered and the bottom or involved leg comfortably bent and lying on the table).

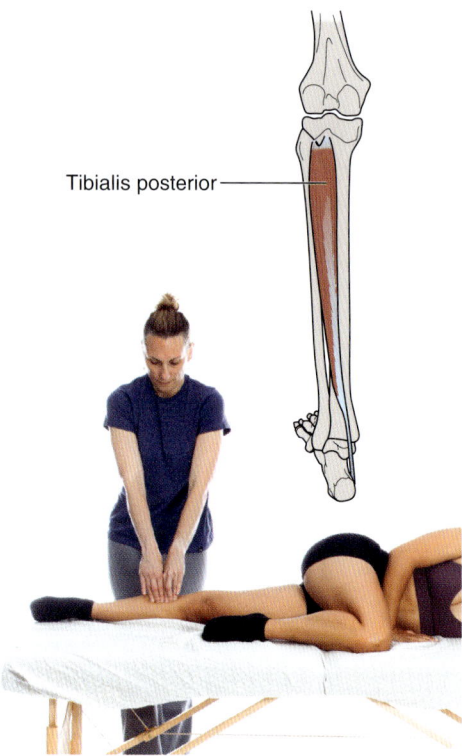

Figure 10.11 Treatment to the deep posterior compartment involves sinking braced fingers just posterior to the tibia on the medial side of the lower leg.

Effective treatment is done posteriorly to the medial aspect of the tibia. It is difficult to perform glides on these muscles based on their location; therefore, the treatment is more static. Sinking your fingertips into the posterior aspect of the tibia and holding a static treatment is very effective. Make sure your fingertips are braced to provide support and your fingernails are trimmed. To add movement, have the patient slowly move between plantar flexion and dorsiflexion or between inversion and eversion. Active engagement is best here to allow you to use braced fingers. As the muscle and fascia start to release, your fingertips will sink more into the tissue. The static hold can start distally and move proximally along the length of the tibia.

Cautions Around the Medial Malleolus

Be cautious when working directly posterior to the medial malleolus where the tibial artery, vein, and nerve sit between the tendons. Also be sure to perform this treatment with short, clean fingernails to avoid breaking the skin or spreading pathogens harbored under the fingernails.

INTRINSIC MUSCLES OF THE FOOT

Four layers of muscles on the plantar surface of the foot are deep to the plantar fascia. Isolation of the muscles is not necessary for treatment purposes, but it is interesting to note which muscles are where. On the dorsal surface of the foot, there is one layer of muscle. In addition, there are muscles between the metatarsals. Most of the muscles are named for their location and function, as described next.

Layers 1 and 2
Adductor hallucis, flexor digitorum brevis, and abductor digiti minimi

Quadratus plantae, lumbricals, flexor digitorum longus tendon, and flexor hallucis longus tendon

Layers 3 and 4
Flexor hallucis brevis

Adductor hallucis oblique head and transverse head

Flexor digiti minimi plantar interossei (three)

Posterior tibialis tendon

Peroneus longus tendon

The dorsal muscles include the dorsal interossei (four), extensor hallucis brevis, and extensor digitorum brevis.

Foot Treatment

Typically, dorsal surface treatment is done with the patient supine and you, the clinician, either seated or standing comfortably. Warming the area can begin with either gentle glides (lower level of pressure) or some compression. Treatment for the dorsal surface can include thumb glides along and between the metatarsals. To support the fingers, used braced thumbs. These glides can include movement of the phalanges.

Treatment for the plantar surface of the foot can be done with the client either supine or prone, depending on the work being done. It is important to maintain your balance, so a seated position may be warranted. Warming the area can start with compressions and even wringing of the foot done by grasping the foot and moving the hands back and forth in opposite directions, squeezing and releasing the foot. Myofascial glides using a loose fist are very effective. Using a loose fist will help decrease the pressure on the finger joints. Extending the toes while gliding can add movement to the treatment. If the client is supine, the correct biomechanics would be gliding from the phalanges to the calcaneus. If the person is prone, the glides can be done from calcaneus to toes. To save your own mechanics, avoid using unbraced fingers or thumbs. Additionally, instead of pushing your fingers into the plantar fascia, place your thumb or the fingers of one hand on the plantar surface of the client's foot, and place your other hand on the dorsal surface of the client's foot. Then you can push the foot (using plantar flexion or plantar flexion with inversion and eversion) into the treating thumb or fingers. To save the thumb, brace with the index finger of the same hand or use two fingers together.

WHY DOES THE CLINICIAN CARE?

From Achilles tendinosis to medial tibial stress syndrome, calf cramps, and ankle sprains, the lower leg can benefit from treatment to the myofascial structures. As the foot hits the ground, the rest of the kinetic chain must adjust (imagine slipping on ice or a wet spot on the floor, and think about how the rest of the body reacts to adjust the center of gravity and prevent a fall). Therefore, treating areas of concern in the low leg can help diminish pain up the kinetic chain that might be compensating for the low leg. Lower-extremity overuse injuries, in particular, favor massage therapy work along with appropriate stretching and strengthening.

Self-Care

As seen in the previous chapters, one manual therapy treatment cannot solve it all. Many of the conditions that clinicians see in athletes are a result of hours of training, poor everyday habits, or muscle response to stress. A balance of stretching and strengthening is needed, addressing postural and phasic responses appropriately. In some cases, muscle stresses cannot be fixed because they are necessary for the sport. Plus, the treatments presented in this book are not meant to be done daily. Most clinicians do not see their clients every day, and even those who do (e.g., athletic trainers) understand that providing only manual therapy daily is not the most efficient option. To make a difference, clinicians must consider what the patient does between sessions and which self-care treatments the patient should use in addition to manual therapy.

Here is an important point of note regarding massage, manual therapy, and all of the adjunct devices included in this chapter: Clinicians should be aware that much of the peer-reviewed literature centers around performance measures. In research, performance measures are easy to capture and are of interest; however, the modalities are not designed as part of performance improvement. When the research design does not match the intent of the product, the outcome will not be statistically significant. Any improvements in performance may also be more clinically relevant to the athlete while not being statistically significant in the research world. In the end, manual therapy work is about feeling better, helping the muscles function better, and decreasing potential injury risks from overuse or biomechanical insufficiencies. Performance improvements are secondary.

Compressive Massage

This discussion refers to any type of myofascial release that falls under the category of compressive massage, including foam rollers, massage sticks, massage canes (e.g., TheraCane), and intermittent compression devices. Remembering the properties of tensegrity from chapter 1, clinicians use compression to adjust the pull on the fascia. With that in mind, do not necessarily just foam roll over an area that feels tight. Consistent compression may compound the area of concern by producing additional soreness and inflammation. One such example is the area of the iliotibial (IT) band where it crosses the lateral femoral condyle. Under the fascia is a fat pad that is highly innervated. Consistent compression over this area can actually lead to increased pain and potentially more inflammation as well. By shifting the foam roller to a spot away from this sensitive area, including stopping superior to the condyle or even shifting the rolling to the medial aspect of the thigh, the clinician can use the principles of tensegrity to shift the fascia in another spot, thereby releasing the fascia at the distal IT band.

Foam Rollers

Foam rolling is a form of self-myofascial release performed using a roller of varying levels of foam density (figure 11.1). This technique is commonly used for warm-up and recovery. The person doing the rolling controls the pressure; they can vary the amount of body weight they put through the area while rolling back and forth over the foam roller. There are no set protocols for foam rolling as far as time, duration, and depth of pressure (Kerautret et al. 2020). Foam rolling is ideal for practitioners to prescribe for patients to do on their own, provided practitioners demonstrate correct techniques and offer feedback as they would with any other therapeutic intervention. Foam rolling is also an effective home care option for clients to use between manual therapy sessions. However, in some cases, people will self-prescribe foam rolling without understanding when compression is desired versus when other techniques would better serve their goals. It is also common for competitive individuals to take a more-is-better approach; with foam rolling, more is definitely not better.

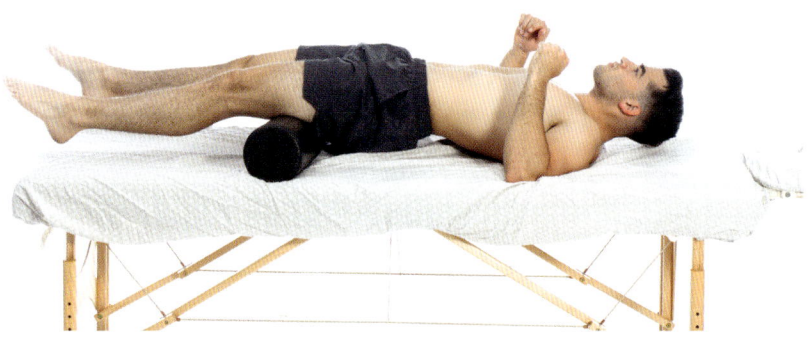

Figure 11.1 The athlete is using his body weight and leverage to create pressure as he uses the foam roller along his hamstrings.

Massage Sticks

Use of a *massage stick* is another form of self-compression of the myofascial areas. This tool features rolling pieces along the length of the stick. Instead of providing compression through body weight, as is done with the foam roller, the massage stick is rolled over the area, with the force coming from the hands or arms. Using the stick requires some level of flexibility to reach the intended areas, which may be self-limiting. Additionally, the ability to generate force is less than when an individual uses their body weight over the device. Because less force is generated, however, the massage stick may be better for someone who tends to overdo the pressure or cannot get into the correct positions to foam roll.

Massage Canes

A *massage cane* (e.g., TheraCane) is a rigid plastic tool with several round knobs, including one knob on the end of the cane and multiple knobs on bars along the shaft (figure 11.2). This tool is used for compression into more concentrated areas of muscle. Whereas the massage stick or foam roller is used to alleviate fascia in a larger area, the massage cane is meant to target specific knots or trigger points through concentrated compression. As with the other techniques mentioned earlier, there are no set time or pressure protocols for the massage cane. It is important to educate clients using this tool (a) to work within their own pain tolerance and (b) to avoid creating bruises or using too much pressure over bony areas, such as the spinous processes. As with all other devices described in this chapter, more pressure and more treatments are not necessarily better. It may be best for

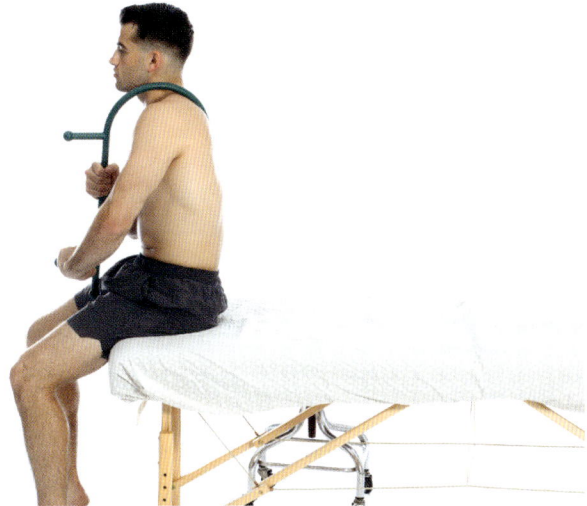

Figure 11.2 The athlete uses a massage cane to reach a knot or trigger point in his upper back.

clinicians to advise patients on when not to use the massage cane, depending on either the manual therapy treatment the clinician has provided or in conjunction with a competition when it may be counterproductive to perform such a targeted self-care treatment.

Balls

There are a variety of round balls specifically designed and marketed to target areas such as the plantar fascia of the foot or the gluteal region. However, there is nothing special about these tools compared to using readily available balls, such as a golf ball for the foot or a lacrosse ball for the gluteal region and hips. Like the massage cane, the ball is used for more specific areas in which there is a knot in the muscle, and it can also be rolled along the area of fascial restriction. Some people may also keep a ball at their desk and do some compression throughout their workday while seated. As with all of the techniques described here, care should be taken not to do too much or use too much pressure.

Intermittent Compression

Intermittent compression includes the use of pneumatic compression via an external unit. Typically, sleeves are applied around the extremity and inflated to a specific pressure to facilitate fluid movement. Although these devices have been used both with and without cold therapy in the clinic to control or reduce swelling, there is little research to support clinical protocols. Postexercise use of recovery boots to reduce fatigue has become more prevalent in the last decade; however, the research on their effects is limited (Prentice 2024). Because the aforementioned devices are general treatments for the limb, they would not be effective in treating specific targeted areas, although they may have overall effects similar to the compressive techniques of massage.

Decompression

Fascial decompression is a technique used to build space within the layers of the fascia. The fascial layers are lifted from the underlying tissues, which allows the layers to slide while also allowing for an increase in fluid into the area. Fluid brings in nutrients and oxygen while allowing for unused materials to return to the circulation. Lifting of the fascia can also allow for greater movement and motion.

Tape

Various brands of *kinesiology tape* (e.g., Kinesio Tape, RockTape, and KT Tape) are all designed to serve as a source of fascial decompression. This type of tape is different from traditional athletic tape, because it is not meant to support the joint or prevent range of motion. Kinesiology tape is not intended to be pulled tight across the skin or provide compression. Regardless of which brand is preferred, the tape is meant to lift the skin, opening spaces in the superficial fascia to allow for fluid movement. Taping falls under the concept of decompression, but it also can elicit feedback from proprioceptors (e.g., Golgi tendon organs and muscle spindle fibers), which can help improve movement. Taping an area after a fascial treatment can potentially help the fascia maintain the new integrity created by the treatment.

Cupping

Cupping is a form of myofascial decompression (figure 11.3). The cups use a vacuum effect to create a negative pressure, increasing blood flow in the immediate area (Wang et al. 2023). In addition to altering blood flow dynamics, the change in pressure can potentially increase erythrocytes and activate the neuroendocrine immune system (Wang et al. 2023). Cupping also is perceived to induce relaxation on a systemic level.

When cupping is taken in the context of fascial therapy, the decompression can help to alleviate the pull of the fascia based on the forces applied. The vacuum creates a pull on the fascia that initiates the forces of tensegrity to redirect the stress on the muscle. Think of the stress applied to the area as a push and the force of the cupping as a pull, returning the fascia to a more appropriate state. Cupping with movement is another way to work within the positive parameters of fascial change.

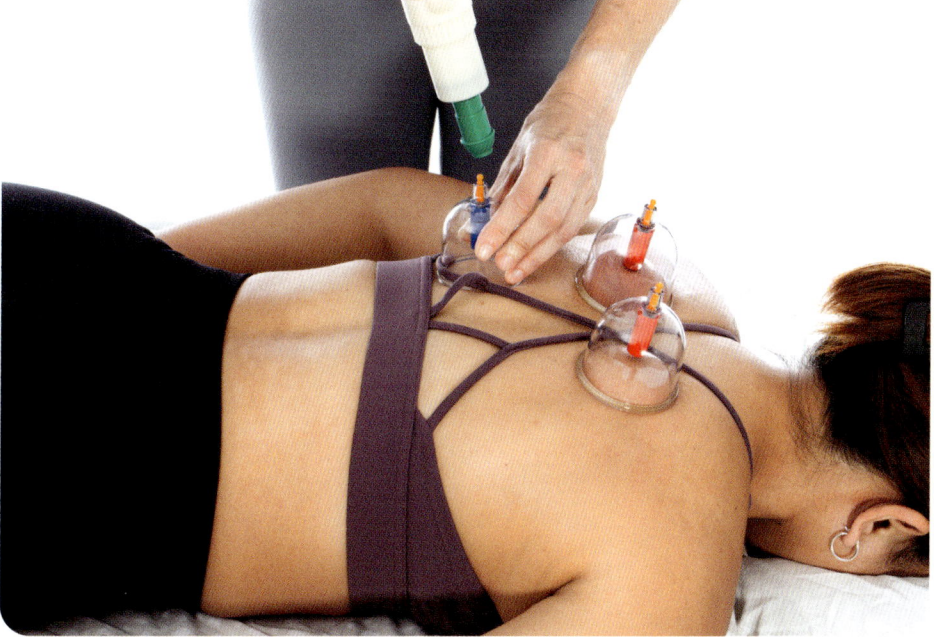

Figure 11.3 Cups are placed along areas of the upper back; air is suctioned out to create negative pressure, increasing the space below the surface of the skin and allowing blood flow to increase in the area.

Percussive Massage

Percussive massage uses vibration in any form applied to the myofascial system (figure 11.4). In a Swedish or relaxation massage, percussion or tapotement is applied using the hands (hacking, beating, or cupping). The vibrating massage chair, often seen in airports or salons, is another form of percussive massage. However, the popularity of massage guns has made percussive treatment readily available and often seen on the sidelines of sporting events. Other forms of percussive massage include the addition of vibration to foam rollers or massage balls to create a compressive device that also provides percussion.

As described in chapter 3, percussive therapies have the same tissue response as the manual percussion techniques described, specifically with regard to fascial and nervous system responses. Percussive therapies can be used to decrease pain, especially the pain of delayed-onset muscle soreness (Sams et al. 2023). This type of treatment can increase blood flow, available oxygen, and tissue temperature, which may contribute to improved metabolic activity (Ferreira et al. 2023). Physiologically, the muscles will relax via reciprocal inhibition and excitation of the muscle spindles (Sams et al. 2023; Ferreira et al. 2023). The Pacinian corpuscles respond to the vibration, eliciting a response from the nervous system (Ferreira et al. 2023).

In research, the use of percussion in various forms has shown an increase in range of motion (Cheatham et al. 2019). The biggest difference in the treatment is the type of device and its portability and ease of use.

Massage Guns

Massage guns provide percussive therapy from a convenient handheld source. Several manufacturers produce these devices; however, all have similar effects. Massage guns usually include a variety of heads that can be attached. Smaller

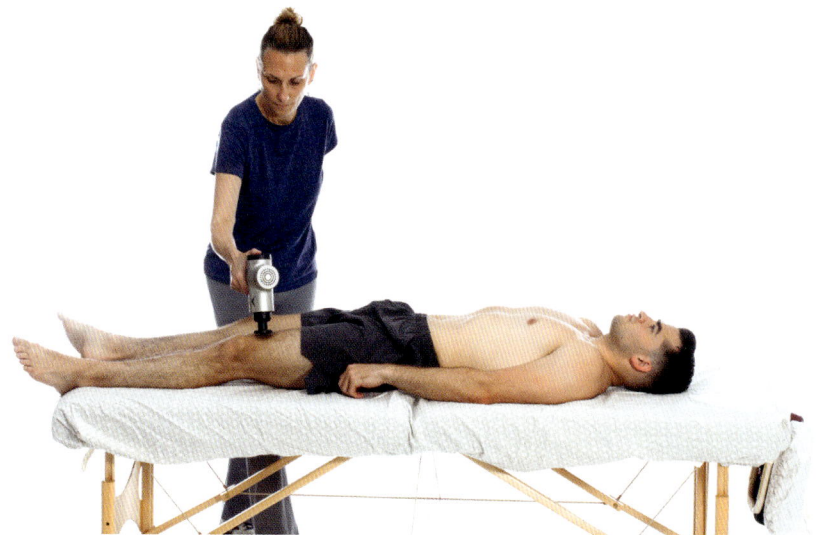

Figure 11.4 The clinician uses a massage gun to provide percussive therapy to the quadriceps.

heads provide a more concentrated treatment. Other options include flat or rounded heads. Depending on the device type, there may be a variety of speeds. Slower speeds are advised for more sensitive areas and areas with less muscle bulk (e.g., the anterior lower leg), whereas faster speeds can be used on more muscular areas (e.g., the thigh).

It is not necessary to push the head of the massage gun into the area, because it is intended to float along the surface. Faster speeds can be used to create the illusion of deeper pressure. The device is intended to continuously move across the muscle belly, with stops focused on the origin and insertion of the muscle. It is important to ensure the gun is moving over the area and not held steady for too long over one spot. Ideally, approximately 30 seconds over each muscle is sufficient, making the massage gun perfect for use during athletic events or when there is a small window for treatment.

Vibrating Foam Rollers

Vibrating foam rollers combine the effects of a percussive tool with the compressive effects of a foam roller. The viscoelastic properties of fascia influenced by compression, in combination with the relaxation and pain-reducing effect of percussion, can be used to positively affect range of motion (Cheatham et al. 2019). The vibrating foam roller comes in ball or roller form and can be used with or without vibration, which makes for a multitasking tool that can be used for different interactions.

Massage Chairs

Massage chairs have built-in mechanisms to apply percussion to different areas of the body. Some massage chairs may add elements of heat to the body as well. Although massage chairs can promote relaxation and have the same benefits seen with other techniques, they should be used with caution. Too much pressure or prolonged use can increase, rather than decrease, muscle soreness. These chairs are not designed to be used for hours on end. The recommended time limit is 15 minutes. For many, the cost and size of the massage chair may outweigh the benefits of having such a luxury in the home.

Hydrotherapy

Hydrotherapy includes any modality that uses water as a medium, which has varying effects on the body systems. The use of water includes its various forms—liquid, solid (ice), and gas (steam)—with internal or external application. Hydrotherapy can be used to increase range of motion, reduce the subjective feelings of delayed-onset muscle soreness, and increase perception of recovery (Mooventhan and Nivethitha 2014). Exercise in an aquatic environment can be beneficial for individuals who can better accommodate exercise with the assistance of buoyancy. Hydrotherapy may be beneficial for individuals who require a reduction of force on the joints, owing to either weight-bearing restrictions in rehabilitation or increased body mass (e.g., obesity).

Individual differences between heat and cold and their various forms are outlined next. As new modalities emerge in this context, it is important to consider the basic physiological responses to hydrotherapy as well as the indications, contraindications, and type of treatment (Mooventhan and Nivethitha 2014).

Cryotherapy

For the purposes of this book, *cryotherapy* includes any use of cold applied either after injury or as a recovery modality. Cooling works not by having the cold modality cool the body, but by the modality pulling the warmth from the body in an effort to equalize temperature. Consider this example: When you put ice in your drink, the ice does not cool the drink; the drink warms the ice. The cooling effect is dependent on the amount of water in the tissue, with tissues with higher water content being excellent conductors of cold and those with lower water content being less effective. Although this cooling effect is true of tissue type (e.g., muscle versus fat), it also may be true of an individual's hydration state. Superficial cold application lowers local metabolic function, decreases muscle spasm, and has an analgesic effect (Mooventhan and Nivethitha 2014). These effects make cold appealing as a recovery modality after a challenging workout, for example, as a way to decrease delayed-onset muscle soreness. Although cold immersion does not decrease metabolic rate (which is a systemic measure, as opposed to a local measure of metabolic function), it decreases heart rate and diastolic blood pressure (Mooventhan and Nivethitha 2014). Vascular changes occur in the area local to the application of cold, with vasodilation occurring to increase blood flow to the area (Mooventhan and Nivethitha 2014). Nerve conduction changes occur, including decreased amplitude and reduced sensory conduction (Mooventhan and Nivethitha 2014). Immersion in a cold tub is also indicated to reduce body temperature in someone who may be experiencing exercise-induced heat illness.

COLD-WATER OR ICE-WATER IMMERSION

An ice bath involves immersion of a body part in a water or ice solution at 50 to 60 degrees Fahrenheit (10-15 °C). The submersion typically lasts 10 to 15 minutes and is ideal for providing cooling around the circumference of the body part. Therapeutically, *cold-water immersion* and *ice-water immersion* have the same benefits as an ice bag, but they also have the advantage of being able to surround the body part and the disadvantage of having the limb in a dependent position.

COLD PLUNGE AND WHOLE-BODY CRYOTHERAPY

Cold plunge and whole-body cryotherapy are two different concepts that overlap somewhat. A *cold plunge* is a full-body immersion in cold water, whereas *whole-body cryotherapy* includes exposure to compressed refrigerated air in an enclosed room to cool the entire body with liquid nitrogen released in the chamber. On a systemic level, cold immersion increases heart rate, blood pressure, and metabolism while decreasing cerebral blood flow depending on the temperature of the immersion (Mooventhan and Nivethitha 2014). Carbon dioxide–enriched water immersion can increase parasympathetic activity. Proposed benefits include decreased pain, fatigue, and muscle soreness as well as an increased feeling of well-being (Mooventhan and Nivethitha 2014). Although this treatment does not have a lot of evidence behind it, there is anecdotal support.

ICE MASSAGE

Ice massage involves the use of water in its solid form as a block applied directly to the skin surface (figure 11.5). This treatment differs from that with a typical ice bag: With ice bag treatment, there is a layer separating the ice from the skin as well as air between the ice cubes. In ice massage, the ice is rubbed over the skin in overlapping circles. Ice massage is indicated for myofascial trigger points, and it can be used to create an analgesic effect before engaging in stretching or exercise.

Thermotherapy

Thermotherapy involves the application of heat to treat disease and injury. The physiological effect of thermotherapy occurs when the heat is absorbed into the tissue and spreads to the adjacent tissue. The type of heat applied, the duration, and the tissue type all factor into the body's response. Heat increases the extensibility of collagen, which is found in connective tissue such as

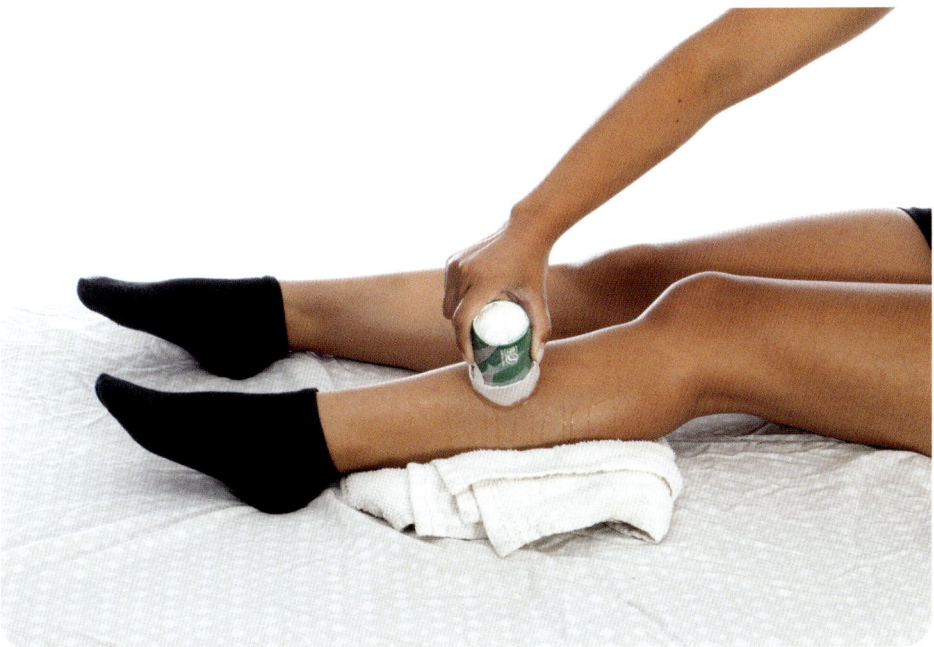

Figure 11.5 The patient performs an ice massage treatment prior to dance rehearsal.

the fascia (Mooventhan and Nivethitha 2014). Using thermotherapy before manual therapy can prewarm the tissues, whereas using it during treatment can enhance techniques that rely on extensibility of the tissues. Additionally, heat can be used to increase blood flow to an ischemic area of muscle, which may relieve muscle guarding. Along with increasing the extensibility of the tendons, heat can be used before stretching for a more effective outcome on range of motion.

HOT PACKS
Many therapeutic settings have a *hydrocollator*, which heats and stores silicate gel–containing hot packs submerged in water held at 160 to 170 degrees Fahrenheit (71.1-76.7 °C). Some commercially available hot packs may also be heated using other elements. The most common indication for these packs is general relaxation and reduction of the pain-spasm-pain cycle. From a massage perspective, hot packs can be used to warm the fascia before treatment; however, the induction of relaxation increases the parasympathetic response, which may not be warranted in all massage treatments (see chapter 2).

HOT TUBS
Hot tubs with jets, or *whirlpools*, involve the combination of water immersion and compressive massage. The effects of thermotherapy and compression lead to relaxation of muscle spasm and decreased pain.

SAUNAS
Although saunas typically are considered a type of hydrotherapy, they may involve steam or more of a dry heat. One example is infrared sauna exposure as a form of full-body thermotherapy. Sauna exposure can increase epinephrine levels (Mooventhan and Nivethitha 2014). Concern with saunas includes overheating if the person is not well hydrated or has a contraindication in which they are unable to dissipate heat well. Saunas should not be used for weight control or to intentionally dehydrate the body.

Additional Self-Care

As discussed earlier, massage alone is not the only key to self-care and works best with adjunct therapies. Stretching and strengthening are two keys to maintaining the benefits of massage. There are also other ways in which people can assist the body in recovery. Although many of these additional self-care approaches are outside the scope of this text and adequately covered in other books, the two that best apply here are hydration and sleep.

Hydration

Fascia likes fluid and fluid movement. Clinicians who have tried to pick up the superficial fascia, such as with taking skinfold measurements or applying the skin rolling technique, might notice how difficult this can be on some people or on some areas of the body. Much of what is experienced in myofascial pain comes from the fascia being adhered to the layers below. Increasing blood flow on a local level is one of the keys to many treatments; however, without enough fluid in the body, there is less fluid to create plasma and interstitial fluid. Although being well hydrated will not stop the fascial system from having issues, it can assist in the recovery process.

There is a fallacy in manual therapy that treatments release toxins from the body and that drinking water will help flush toxins from the system. There is no research or scientific support to this claim, yet it is perpetuated among clinicians and the public. The human body has the liver for detoxification and the kidneys to eliminate waste products. Muscle soreness can come from the release of myofascial trigger points; however, the body's response is similar to that found with delayed-onset muscle soreness. Regardless, staying hydrated, in general and after a treatment, is a good thing.

Sleep

Sleep is the body's time to repair. Adequate sleep is another key to aid the recovery process. Sleep deprivation can lead to decreases in cognition, memory, and motor skills and can also negatively affect mental health. During sleep, the body uses the time to repair muscles, bones, and joints and to recover from the stresses of the day. Benefits of adequate sleep include feelings of happiness, regulation of hunger hormones, increased productivity, and strengthening of the immune system. Research into athletic performance shows impaired reaction time when an athlete is sleep deprived and improved performance on skills with adequate sleep (Kirschen et al. 2018).

Because negative stress leads to sleep issues such as insomnia, creating a more relaxed atmosphere can help aid in sleep. Using manual therapy to promote parasympathetic dominance can assist in relaxation, hence leading to better sleep. If sleep promotion is the goal, a more relaxing massage can be done later in the day, closer to bedtime. However, if the goals of the session align with techniques that might produce more of a sympathetic response, the timing of the treatment might be better earlier in the day or before activity. Just as timing and treatment choices are important in relation to activity, they also are important in relation to sleep and recovery.

What the Pros Are Doing and Why

Professional athletes often have access to modalities that are either cost-prohibitive or otherwise unavailable to the public. Additionally, full-time professional athletes have more time and more resources to seek out these treatments. Although the physiological starting point for these athletes is ahead of the public, they, too, have physiological limits. Even with all the best resources available, it is physiologically impossible to speed up healing time or to physiologically increase the body's ability to gain fitness or strength beyond its limits. However, all individuals, athletes and nonathletes alike, can provide an optimal environment for these changes to occur. Examples including hydration, rest (in the form of sleep, but also in the form of days off from training or adjustments to training, including substituting yoga or stretching for a cardiorespiratory or strength workout), and paying attention to nutritional needs.

What Athletes Should Avoid

The idea behind this section is myth versus reality, because there are some things athletes absolutely should not do. There are numerous myths about what does and does not work. Although clinicians cannot change everyone's mind, they can provide patient education and tools to help people make good decisions. As important as it is for clinicians to be educated in the types of treatment, it is equally as important for them to educate the athletes they are working with as to what treatments they should and should not be doing on their own.

Manual therapy is one area in which clinicians who are unsure of the *why* behind a treatment will often let the patient receiving the treatment dictate care. Although patient-centered care is important and buy-in is paramount, providing a treatment that lacks scientific merit or is counter to the goals based on physiological responses is irresponsible. As pointed out with hydration earlier, massage does not release toxins from the tissues; therefore, using massage to release chemicals does not have a physiological basis. Massage cannot be used to break up cellulite or melt fat; treatments cannot assist in gaining muscle. Like many other modalities, the goal of manual therapy is to put the body in an optimal position to perform, even if performance measures do not improve.

When compressive techniques such as foam rolling are used, the treatment duration should be limited, as should the pressure. There is no more-is-better approach: Too much pressure can inhibit the desired response and even cause bruising and pain. If a self-treatment is not resulting in change, the clinician should assess the situation, ensure the patient is performing the prescribed self-treatment correctly, and then determine whether an alternate treatment would be better. As pointed out earlier, care should be taken in specific body regions (e.g., the distal IT band), owing to pain receptors in those areas. Eliciting more pain will cause the tissue to guard more and not release. Also, continuing to roll over a bruised area can cause more pain and potentially inflammation in the area. If the issue is continued trigger points or tight areas, stretching the postural muscles and strengthening the phasic muscles may provide the relief the client seeks. As noted earlier, a more-is-better approach is not always best when it comes to these treatments.

Treatments should be done in relation to training goals and performance goals. Here is where patient-centered care comes into play, with the clinician informing the patient of the appropriate time to do a treatment. Treatments do not need to be done every day. For example, trigger point release, which can be painful, might be warranted once a week or even less frequently. Treatments that are more relaxing should not be done immediately before practice or competition.

Compressive treatments should not follow decompressive treatments. If the goal of a particular workout is maximal effort, soreness will occur. Therefore, using manual therapy, especially compressive techniques, might be counterintuitive because it could compound the soreness.

Part of training involves increasing demand to make gains, and treatments should be used to help patients achieve their goals rather than impede their progress. For example, the self-care techniques described in this chapter may be better served on a recovery day than daily or after an intense workout or not be used after an intense workout. It is also important for clients to use these self-care techniques correctly. Clinicians can help by demonstrating proper use and correcting clients as needed.

Contraindications and Treatment Safety

General contraindications that apply to the massage techniques in this book are listed in chapter 3. However, there are more to consider when applying some of the additional self-care therapies described here, and it is important for clinicians to share these safety tips with clients who will use a device or treatment on their own.

With shared objects such as cups or instruments, it is important to adequately clean these items to prevent the spread of pathogens. It also is important for individuals with a skin pathogen to avoid using these tools, particularly shared items such as foam rollers or percussive guns.

Varicose veins are listed as a caution site for manual therapy, which is especially important when using a percussive instrument or intermittent compression. Blood can pool at the site of the varicosity, potentially creating a clot. The aforementioned treatments could dislodge the clot and move it into the systemic circulation.

Cleanliness is also paramount when using hydrotherapy tubs, hot packs that may be shared (including the covers), and foam rollers, which are often left out for anyone to use. Even something as simple as placing a towel over the skin or requiring postpractice showers can be beneficial. Because the majority of this text is only centered around musculoskeletal issues, readers are advised to consult pathology texts for specifics on when certain manual therapy treatments would be contraindicated for illnesses (see Werner 2019).

WHY DOES THE CLINICIAN CARE?

It is important to note that much of the research performed and cited surrounding the self-care therapies described in this chapter is not necessarily done in the context of clinical practice. Many times, the outcome measures used in research are performance measures. None of these treatments in isolation can make someone run faster or jump higher. Smaller studies tend to show no significant difference between the treatment and a control or sham, either because of the small subject pool or the small effect size of the treatment. With systematic reviews and meta-analyses, often it is hard to combine studies because of a lack of continuity in treatment protocols, which is another important consideration for clinicians reading the research. Most studies do not provide a methodology that is applicable to the intended effects of the treatment, nor do they align with a clinical practice. Clinicians would argue that they cannot use a set manual therapy protocol in the clinical setting; therefore, following the protocol established in research would not allow for duplication. An evidence-based clinician thus is encouraged to use the device based on the type of treatment it will provide and not based solely on the results of a strict research protocol.

Although this book may not be updated as quickly as hot self-care trends and devices arrive on the market, the principles outlined here are intended to stand the test of time. Any new form of stick or foam roller would fall under the category of compressive techniques, as would a massage cane or a type of instrument-assisted treatment. In this case, the fascial change comes from the application of pressure, working with the properties of tensegrity. Options such as kinesiology tape and cupping are types of decompressive techniques, in which fluid movement is encouraged. Keeping the balance of the technique's intent is key to helping its effects last longer. For example, if the desired effect is decompression, it would be ill-advised to do a cupping treatment prior to foam rolling.

Bibliography

Archer, P.A. 2007. *Therapeutic massage in athletics*. LWW Massage Therapy and Bodywork Educational Series. Philadelphia: Lippincott Williams & Wilkins.

Biel, A. 2019. *Trail guide to movement: Building the body in motion*. 2nd ed. Boulder, CO: Books of Discovery.

Bini, R.R., and A. Flores Bini. 2018. Potential factors associated with knee pain in cyclists: A systematic review. *Open Access Journal of Sports Medicine* 9: 99-106. https://doi.org/10.2147/OAJSM.S136653.

Cambron, J.A., J. Dexheimer, and P. Coe. 2006. Changes in blood pressure after various forms of therapeutic massage: A preliminary study. *Journal of Alternative and Complementary Medicine* 12(1): 65-70. https://doi.org/10.1089/acm.2006.12.65.

Chaitow, L., and J. DeLany. 2000. *Clinical application of neuromuscular technique*. 2 vols. Edinburgh: Churchill Livingstone.

Cheatham, S.W., K.R. Stull, and M.J. Kolber. 2019. Comparison of a vibration roller and a nonvibration roller intervention on knee range of motion and pressure pain threshold: A randomized controlled trial. *Journal of Sport Rehabilitation* 28(1): 39-45. https://doi.org/10.1123/jsr.2017-0164.

Choi, T.Y., L. Ang, B. Ku, J.H. Jun, and M.S. Lee. 2021. Evidence map of cupping therapy. *Journal of Clinical Medicine* 10(8): 1750. https://doi.org/10.3390/jcm10081750.

Ferreira, R.M., R. Silva, P. Vigario, P.N. Martins, F. Casanova, R.J. Fernandes, and A.R. Sampaio. 2023. The effects of massage guns on performance and recovery: A systematic review. *Journal of Functional Morphology and Kinesiology* 8(3): 138. https://doi.org/10.3390/jfmk8030138.

Floyd, R.T. 2015. *Manual of structural kinesiology*. 19th ed. New York: McGraw Hill Education.

Fritz, S. 2017. *Mosby's fundamentals of therapeutic massage*. 6th ed. St. Louis, MO: Elsevier.

Houglum, P.A. 2016. *Therapeutic exercise for musculoskeletal injuries*. 4th ed. Champaign, IL: Human Kinetics.

Kerautret, Y., F. Di Rienzo, C. Eyssautier, and A. Guillot. 2020. Selective effects of manual massage and foam rolling on perceived recovery and performance: Current knowledge and future directions toward robotic massages. *Frontiers in Physiology* 11: 598898. https://doi.org/10.3389/fphys.2020.598898.

Kirschen G.W., J.J. Jones, and L. Hale. 2018. The impact of sleep duration on performance among competitive athletes: A systematic literature review. *Clinical Journal of Sport Medicine*.

Konrad, A., C. Glashuttner, M.M. Reiner, D. Bernsteiner, and M. Tilp. 2020. The acute effects of a percussive massage treatment with a hypervolt device on plantar flexor muscles' range of motion and performance. *Journal of Sports Science and Medicine* 19(4): 690-694. www.ncbi.nlm.nih.gov/pubmed/33239942.

Kumka, M., and J. Bonar. 2012. Fascia: A morphological description and classification system based on a literature review. *Journal of the Canadian Chiropractic Association* 56(3): 179-191. www.ncbi.nlm.nih.gov/pubmed/22997468.

Loghmani, M., and M. Whitted. 2016. Soft tissue manipulation: A powerful form of mechanotherapy. *Journal of Physiotherapy & Physical Rehabilitation* 1(4): 1000122. https://doi.org/10.4172/2573-0312.1000122.

Mayes, M., M. Salesky, and D.A. Lansdown. 2022. Throwing injury prevention strategies with a whole kinetic chain-focused approach. *Current Reviews in Musculoskeletal Medicine* 15(2): 53-64. https://doi.org/10.1007/s12178-022-09744-9.

Moore, K.L., A.M.R. Agur, and A.F. Dalley. 2011. *Essential clinical anatomy*. 4th ed. Baltimore, MD: Lippincott Williams & Wilkins.

Mooventhan, A., and L. Nivethitha. 2014. Scientific evidence-based effects of hydrotherapy on various systems of the body. *North American Journal of Medicine and Science* 6(5): 199-209. www.ncbi.nlm.nih.gov/pubmed/24926444.

Moraska, A. 2005. Sports massage. A comprehensive review. *Journal of Sports Medicine and Physical Fitness* 45(3): 370-380. www.ncbi.nlm.nih.gov/pubmed/16230990.

Nicola, T.L., and D.J. Jewison. 2012. The anatomy and biomechanics of running. *Clinics in Sports Medicine* 31(2): 187-201. https://doi.org/10.1016/j.csm.2011.10.001.

Poppendieck, W., M. Wegmann, A. Ferrauti, M. Kellmann, M. Pfeiffer, and T. Meyer. 2016. Massage and performance recovery: A meta-analytical review. *Sports Medicine* 46(2): 183-204. https://doi.org/10.1007/s40279-015-0420-x.

Prentice, W.E. 2024. *Principles of athletic training: A guide to evidence-based clinical practice*. New York: McGraw Hill.

Resnick, P.B. 2016. Comparing the effects of rest and massage on return to homeostasis following submaximal aerobic exercise: A case study. *International Journal of Therapeutic Massage & Bodywork* 9(1): 4-10. www.ncbi.nlm.nih.gov/pubmed/26977215.

Resnick, P.B. 2024. Ergonomic considerations for practicing massage therapists. *International Journal of Therapeutic Massage & Bodywork* 17(3): 41-47. https://doi.org/10.3822/ijtmb.v17i3.983.

Robertson, D., I. Biaggioni, G. Burnstock, and P.A. Low, eds. 2004. *Primer on the autonomic nervous system*. 2nd ed. San Diego, CA: Elsevier.

Sams, L., B.L. Langdown, J. Simons, and J. Vseteckova. 2023. The effect of percussive therapy on musculoskeletal performance and experiences of pain: A systematic literature review. *International Journal of Sports Physical Therapy* 18(2): 309-327. https://doi.org/10.26603/001c.73795.

Schleip, R. 2003a. Fascial plasticity—A new neurobiological explanation: Part 1. *Journal of Bodywork and Movement Therapies* 7(1): 11-19.

Schleip, R. 2003b. Fascial plasticity—A new neurobiological explanation: Part 2. *Journal of Bodywork and Movement Therapies* 7(2): 104-116.

Stecco, A., F. Giordani, C. Fede, C. Pirri, R. De Caro, and C. Stecco. 2023. From muscle to the myofascial unit: Current evidence and future perspectives. *International Journal of Molecular Sciences* 24(5): 4527. https://doi.org/10.3390/ijms24054527.

Stecco, A., R. Stern, I. Fantoni, R. De Caro, and C. Stecco. 2016. Fascial disorders: Implications for treatment. *PM & R* 8(2): 161-168. https://doi.org/10.1016/j.pmrj.2015.06.006.

Travell, J.G., and D.G. Simons. 1983. *Myofascial pain and dysfunction: The trigger point manual*. 2 vols. Baltimore, MD: Williams & Wilkins.

Wang, L., Z. Cai, X. Li, and A. Zhu. 2023. Efficacy of cupping therapy on pain outcomes: An evidence-mapping study. *Frontiers in Neurology* 14: 1266712. https://doi.org/10.3389/fneur.2023.1266712.

Werner, R. 2019. *A massage therapist's guide to pathology: Critical thinking and practical application*. 7th ed. Boulder, CO: Books of Discovery.

Willard, F.H., A. Vleeming, M.D. Schuenke, L. Danneels, and R. Schleip. 2012. The thoracolumbar fascia: Anatomy, function and clinical considerations. *Journal of Anatomy* 221(6): 507-536. https://doi.org/10.1111/j.1469-7580.2012.01511.x.

Index

A

abdomen
  manual therapies 145-147, 148
  muscles 142-145
  structure 134
abdominal spiraling 146
abductor digiti minimi 110
abductor pollicis brevis 109
abductor pollicis longus 108
acetabulofemoral joint
  adductor actions 162-164
  gluteal muscle actions 170, 174-176
  hamstring actions 159, 160
  quadriceps actions 156
  structural problems 56
  structure 152-153
acetabulum 152-153
acetylcholine 9
Achilles tendinosis 59-60
Achilles tendon 59-60, 191, 194, 195
acromioclavicular joint 75
actin 12
active insufficiency 66
adductor brevis 163
adductor hiatus 164
adductor longus 162-163
adductor magnus 161, 163-164, 167
adductor pollicis 110, 111
agonists 9
all-or-none principle 9
ankle instability 47
ankle sprains 47, 182-183, 189
ankle structure 182-183
annular ligament 78
annulus fibrosis 51
antagonists 10
anterior abdominal region 142-147
anterior cervical muscles 127-129
anterior compartment (lower leg) 181, 185-188
anterior cruciate ligament 47, 154
anterior deltoid 88
anterior inferior iliac spine 173
anterior pelvic tilt 57
anterior superior iliac spine (ASIS) 152, 173, 176-177
anterior talofibular ligament 183
aponeuroses 5, 7, 87, 134-135
arches of foot 183-184
arms
  elbow and radioulnar joint muscles 99-104
  forearm muscles 66-67, 79, 107-109
  manual therapies 105-106, 110-111
  wrist and hand muscles 107-110
arteries, massage cautions 19-20
arthrogenic muscle inhibition 48, 153
ASIS (anterior superior iliac spine) 152, 173, 176-177
asthma 23
atlantoaxial joint 113
atlantooccipital joint 113
atlas 113
autonomic nervous system 24, 25-26, 27
avulsion fractures 164
axial skeleton stressors 70
axiohumeral muscles 86-88
axioscapular muscles 80-85, 115-117
axis 113

B

balls (massage) 204
beating 38
biceps brachii 53-54, 99, 105
biceps femoris 158, 160-161, 168, 169

217

bicipital aponeurosis 5, 7
bipennate arrangements 10
body mechanics for massage 34-35
bone spurs 46
bony landmarks 13-14, 44-45, 60-61
brachialis 100, 105
brachioradialis 101-102
breathing muscles 22, 23-24, 84, 118-119, 129
bursitis 160, 175

C
calcaneofibular ligament 183
calcaneus 46, 59, 181, 182
cancers 41
carbon dioxide–enriched water immersion 209
cardiac muscle 9
cardiovascular system 18-20, 21, 27
carpal bones 78
carpometacarpal joints 108
cervical muscles 119-121, 127-129
cervical spine 113-114
chronic ankle instability 47
circle of Willis 126
circulatory systems 18-21
circulatory treatments 29-30
cleanliness 198, 213
coccyx 133
cocking phase of throwing 65
cold plunge 208-209
cold-water immersion 208
compressions
  contraindications 188, 212-213
  foot 199
  gluteal region 172-173
  hip 178
  low back 140
  lower leg 193
  in self-care 201-204, 207
  shoulder 93, 96
  technique described 37
  thigh 167, 168
  upper back 121, 132

compressive fascia 5
compressive massage 201-204
concussion 126
contractility 9
contraindications in self-care 212-213
contraindications to massage 41
coracoacromial ligament 75
coracobrachialis 92, 93, 106
coracoclavicular ligaments 75
coracohumeral ligament 75
coracoid process 61
cross-fiber friction 37
cruciate ligaments 154
crural fascia 7
cryotherapy 208-209
cupping 31, 38, 205
cycling 69-70

D
Davis' law 13-14
decompression 31, 204-205
deep fascia, manual therapies for 31
deep posterior compartment (lower leg) 181, 195-198
deep rotators of hip 171-172, 173
deltoids 88, 96
diaphragm 22
diastasis rectus 142-143
disc pathologies 51
distal attachments 11
distal tendon 161
dominant sides of body 16
dorsal interossei 110
drumming 38
dynamic fascia 5

E
edema 20
effleurage 26, 34-35
elasticity 9
elbow
  joint structure 77-78
  manual therapies 105-106
  muscles 9-10, 99-104, 107, 108

performing treatment with 141, 168, 176, 178
  ulnar collateral ligament tear 47-48
emollients 41-42
endomysium 4
epimysium 4, 11
erector spinae group 136-137, 138, 140-141
excitability 9
exhalation 22
expiration 22
extensibility 9
extensor carpi radialis brevis 108, 109
extensor carpi radialis longus 108, 109
extensor carpi ulnaris 108, 109
extensor digiti minimi 108, 109
extensor digitorum 108, 109
extensor digitorum longus 186-187
extensor hallucis longus 187
extensor indicis 108-109
extensor pollicis brevis 108
extensor pollicis longus 108
external obliques 143, 147, 148
extrinsic muscles of wrist and hand 107

F

fascia lata 7, 58-59, 153, 175
fascial decompression 204-205
fascial lines 6
fascia structures and functions 4-7
fascicles 4
femoral nerve 162
femoral triangle 50, 162, 163
femur
  ACL actions on 47, 154
  in knee joint 58, 153
  menisci 48
  muscles 155, 161, 165
  stability in hip joint 49, 152
fibula
  connective tissue 182
  deep posterior compartment 195
  joints 181, 182
  lateral compartment 189, 190
  manual therapy cautions 191
figure-four position 166
first metacarpophalangeal joint 79
flat muscles 10
flexion 151
flexor carpi radialis 107
flexor carpi ulnaris 107
flexor digiti minimi 110
flexor digitorum longus 196-197
flexor digitorum profundus 107, 108
flexor digitorum superficialis 107, 108
flexor hallucis longus 197
flexor pollicis brevis 109
flexor pollicis longus 107
"flush" massage 42
foam rolling 202, 207
focused breathing 22-23
foot 67-69, 183-184, 199
forearm muscles 66-67, 79, 107-109
forward head posture 54
friction technique 37
functional problems
  common knee issues 58-59
  common leg and foot issues 59-60
  common shoulder issues 52-54
  hip joint 56-58
  low back 55-56
  manual therapy's role 51-52
  neck and upper back 54-55
fusiform muscles 10

G

gastrocnemius 191, 192, 193-194
gemellus inferior 172
gemellus superior 172
glenohumeral joint 75-76, 77, 99
glenohumeral ligaments 75
glenoid cavity 49, 75
glenoid labrum 76
gluteal region 170-175
gluteus maximus 170-171

gluteus medius 45, 173, 174, 178
gluteus minimus 173, 174-175, 178
goals for treatment 17, 27, 48, 211, 213
Golgi tendon organs 15
gracilis 164
greater trochanter 175
grip-related stressors 66-67
gutter muscles 137

H
hacking 38
hallux 183
hammer curls 102
hamstrings 158-161, 167-168, 171
hand
  joints 78, 79
  manual therapies 111
  muscles 109-110
heart 18
heat applications 209-210
hemipelvis issues 45
high ankle sprain 183
hip joint
  common functional problems 56, 69
  labral tears 49-50, 152-153
  manual therapies 172-173, 176-179
  manual therapy cautions 166-167, 173
  muscles 153, 155-164, 170-172, 174-176
  shoulder joint versus 151
histamine 19
hot packs 210
hot tubs 210
humeral head 49
humeroulnar joint 77, 78. *See also* elbow
hydration 210-211
hydrocollator packs 210
hydrotherapy 207-210
hyperpronation 60
hypothenar eminence 109, 110, 111

I
ice massage 209
ice-water immersion 208
iliocostalis 136
iliofemoral ligament 152
iliotibial (IT) band
  fascia lata relation to 153, 157, 175
  location and function 6, 7
  manual therapies 178-179
  manual therapy cautions 202
  potential causes of tightness 58-59
  vastus lateralis dysfunction and 157
iliotibial band syndrome 58-59, 179
infraspinatus 90
inguinal ligament 7, 50, 134, 143, 153
inguinal region, avoiding 166-167
inhalation 22
insertions, defined 11
inspiration 22
intercarpal joints 79
intermittent compression 30, 204
internal obliques 144, 147, 148
interosseous membranes 7, 182, 196
interphalangeal joints (foot) 183
interphalangeal joints (hand) 79, 108, 110
intertarsal joints 182, 183
intervertebral discs 51
intrinsic muscles of wrist and hand 107
ischiofemoral ligament 152
isometric contractions 9, 14
isotonic contractions 9
IT band. *See* iliotibial (IT) band

J
Jones fracture 190
jostling 36

K
kind elbow 141, 168, 176, 178
kinesiology tape 204-205
knee joint

anterior cruciate ligament injury 47
common functional problems 58-59
muscles acting on 155-161, 164, 176, 192-193
postsurgery rehabilitation 48-49
structure 153-154
kyphosis 51
kyphotic curves 50, 51

L

labrum injuries
  hip 49-50, 152-153
  shoulder 49, 76, 99
lateral collateral ligament 154
lateral compartment (lower leg) 181, 189-191
lateral epicondyle 109
lateral femoral condyle 202
lateral head of triceps brachii 102, 103
lateral iliac crest 178
lateral longitudinal arch 183
lateral malleolus 189, 190
lateral meniscus 48, 154
lateral pelvic tilt 56
latissimus dorsi 87-88, 96-97
leg length discrepancy 45
legs. See knee joint; lower leg; thigh
levator scapulae 83-84, 117
lift and shift technique 40, 97
ligaments
  ankle 182-183
  common structural issues 46-48
  elbow 78
  foot 183-184
  inguinal 7, 50, 134, 143, 153
  knee joint 153, 154
  pelvis 152, 153
  shoulder 74-75
  wrist 79, 104
ligamentum nuchae 124
linea alba 142-143
local contraindications 41
long head of biceps femoris 160, 161

long head of triceps brachii 102-103
longissimus 136
lordosis 51, 57
lordotic curves 50-51
low back
  causes of pain 55-56, 136, 139-140, 149
  common functional problems 55-56
  manual therapies 140-141, 147-148
  muscles 136-140
  structure 133-134
lower cross syndrome 57
lower leg
  anterior compartment muscles 181, 185-188
  common functional problems 59-60
  deep posterior compartment muscles 181, 195-197
  lateral compartment muscles 181, 189-190
  manual therapies 188, 190-191, 193-195, 197-198
  structure 181-182
  superficial posterior compartment muscles 181, 191-193
lower limb-length inequality 45
lower trapezius 80-81, 115, 122
lubricants 41-42
lumbar spine structure 133-134. See also low back
lumbricals 110
lymphatic system 20-21, 30

M

manual therapies. See also self-care
  abdomen 145-147, 148
  arms 105-106, 110-111
  cardiovascular system effects 18-20
  circulatory treatment types 29-30
  common massage techniques 33-41
  emollients for 41-42
  fallacies about 211, 212
  foot 199

manual therapies (*continued*)
  hand 111
  hip joint 172-173, 176-179
  low back 140-141, 147-148
  lower leg 188, 190-191, 193-195, 197-198
  lymphatic system effects 20, 21
  muscle responses to 32-33
  myofascial treatment overview 30-31
  neck 116, 121-122, 124, 129-132
  nervous system effects 24-26
  respiratory system effects 23-24
  shoulder 49, 93-95, 96-98
  thigh 165-169, 176-179
  upper back 96-97, 121, 123, 132
manual therapy cautions
  Achilles tendon 195
  blood vessels and nerves 19-20, 194, 198
  fibula and peroneal nerve 191
  general concerns 212-213
  gluteal region 173
  inguinal region 166-167
  IT band compression 202
  massage contraindications 41
  medial malleolus 198
  popliteal space 194
  tibia 188
manubrium 74
massage. *See also* manual therapies
  common techniques 33-41
  contraindications 41
  emollients for 41-42
  fallacies about 211, 212
  hot packs with 210
  self-care with 201-204, 206-207
massage canes 203-204
massage chairs 132, 207
massage guns 206-207
massage sticks 203
mastoid process 130
mechanoreceptors 15, 25
medial collateral ligament 154
medial epicondyle 107-108

medial head of triceps brachii 102-103
medial longitudinal arch 183, 184, 196
medial malleolus 195, 197, 198
medial meniscus 48, 154
medial tibial stress syndrome 59, 196
median nerve 104
menisci 48, 153, 154
metacarpal bones 78
metacarpophalangeal joints 79, 108, 110
metatarsal bones 183
metatarsophalangeal joints 183
middle deltoid 88
middle trapezius 80-81, 115, 122
motor units 9
multifidus 138-139, 141
multipennate arrangements 10
muscles. *See also specific muscles*
  basic tissue types and functions 9-10
  fascia connection to 4-5
  physiological principles 13-15, 33, 34
  postural vs. phasic 12-13
  responses to manual therapy 32-33
  shapes and fiber arrangements 4, 10-12
muscle shortening 13, 45
muscle spindle fibers 15
myofascial compression 31, 201-204. *See also* compressions
myofascial decompression 31, 204-205
myofascial glides
  arm 105-106, 110, 111
  foot 199
  hand 111
  low back 140
  lower leg 188, 190, 193
  neck 130-131
  purpose 26
  shoulder 93, 95, 96
  stretching with 41
  technique described 39

    thigh 165-166, 168-169
    upper back 121-122
myofascial release
    avoiding lubricants 41
    overview of techniques 30-31, 38-41
    in postsurgery rehabilitation 47
    self-care techniques 201-207
    with stress fractures 46
myofascial unit 3, 13-15, 34
myofilaments 11-12
myosin 12

N

navicular bone 184
neck
    functional problems 54-55
    manual therapies 116, 121-122,
        124, 129-132
    muscles 115-116, 119-121, 125-129
nervous system overview 24-26
neutralizers 10
nuchal lines 130
nucleus pulposis 51
nursemaid's elbow 78

O

obliquus capitis inferior 126
obliquus capitis superior 125-126
obturator externus 172
obturator internus 172
obturator nerve 162
olecranon 141
olecranon process 168
opponens digiti minimi 110
opponens pollicis 109-110
origins, defined 11
osteitis pubis 164
osteoblasts 46
osteoclasts 46
overhead sports motions 66

P

Pacinian corpuscles 15, 25
palmar interossei 110

palmaris longus 107
parasympathetic nervous system 25-26
passive fascia 5
patella 58, 154, 155
patellofemoral joint 154, 157
patellofemoral pain syndrome 58
pathogens, preventing spread 198, 213
patient-centered care 212, 213
pectineus 162
pectoral fascia 7
pectoralis major 86-87, 93-94
pectoralis minor 84-85, 94-95
pelvis. *See also* hip joint
    bone structure issues 45
    common functional problems
        56-58, 69
    joints 151-153
    manual therapy cautions
        166-167, 173
    muscles 136, 139-140, 155-156,
        158, 174
pennate arrangements 10
percussion techniques 38, 206-207
performance measures 201, 214
performing artists 63-64
perimysium 4
periosteum 11
peroneal nerve 191
peroneus brevis 189-190
peroneus longus 189
peroneus tertius 187-188
pes anserine 59, 160
pes planus 184, 196
petrissage 26, 35-36
phalangeal joints (foot) 183, 187
phalangeal joints (hand) 79, 108-109,
    110
phalanges (foot) 183
phalanges (hand) 78
phasic muscles 12, 13
pin and stretch technique 40-41,
    96-97, 173
piriformis 171, 172, 173
piriformis syndrome 58

plantar aponeurosis 7
plantar calcaneonavicular ligament 184
plantar fascia 6, 7, 184, 199
plantar fasciitis 46, 60
plantar flexion 186, 192
plantaris 191, 192, 193, 194
plasma 20
popliteal space 194
posterior cervical muscles 119-121
posterior cruciate ligament 154
posterior deltoid 88, 96
posterior lumbar region 136-141. *See also* low back
posterior superior iliac spine 141
posterior talofibular ligament 183
posterior tibialis 196
postisometric relaxation 14
postural muscles 12-13
pregnancy 23, 41, 152
pronation of foot 69
pronator quadratus 104, 108
pronator teres 104, 108
proprioception
   ankle instability and 47, 189
   muscles of 118, 119, 126, 185, 189
protracted shoulder 53
proximal attachments 11
pubic symphysis 152
pubofemoral ligament 152

Q
quadratus femoris 172
quadratus lumborum
   lateral pelvic tilt and 56
   leg length inequality and 45
   low back pain and 136
   manual therapies 141, 147-148
   origins, insertions, actions, and innervation 139
   scoliosis and 44
   stressors 139-140
quadratus plantae 197

quadriceps
   functions 155, 158
   manual therapies 165-166
   muscles 155-158
   patellar tracking 58, 154, 155, 156
   rehabilitation 48

R
racket sports 66-67
radiate muscles 10
radioulnar joint 77, 78, 99, 104. *See also* elbow
reciprocal inhibition 14-15, 41
recovery boots 204
rectus abdominis 142-143, 146-147
rectus capitis posterior major 125, 126
rectus capitis posterior minor 125
rectus femoris 155-156, 166, 173
relaxation massage 30, 34-38, 206
research, limitations of 201, 214
respiratory system 22-24
retinacula 7, 188
rhomboids 81-82, 116-117, 122
ribs 114
righting reflex 54, 126
rotator cuff muscles
   dysfunctions 89-90
   functions 49, 89, 90-91
   manual therapies 53, 96
   strengthening programs 82
rotator cuff tears 53
rotatores 138, 139
Ruffini organs 15, 25
running stressors 67-69

S
sacroiliac joint 151-152
sacrospinous ligament 152
sacrotuberous ligament 152
sacrum 133, 151
sarcolemma 4
sarcomeres 11, 12
sartorius 173, 176, 177

saunas 210
scalenes 128-129, 131
scapula
   mispositioning problems 23, 53, 54-55, 82
   movements 76-77
   winging 85
scapular dyskinesis 23-24, 55
scapular protraction 54, 55
scapulohumeral muscles 82, 88-93
scapulohumeral rhythm 66, 77
scapulothoracic joint 73-74, 76-77
sciatica 58
sciatic nerve 58, 172
scoliosis 23, 44-45
self-care
   compressive massage 201-204
   fascial decompression 204-205
   hydrotherapy 207-210
   percussive massage 206-207
   sleep and hydration 210-212
   what to avoid 212-213
semimembranosus 158, 159, 164, 167, 169
semispinalis 121, 138, 139
semitendinosus 158, 159-160, 168, 169
separating fascia 5
serratus anterior 85, 94, 95
serratus posterior inferior 117, 119
serratus posterior superior 117, 118-119, 122-123
shaking 36
shin splints 59, 196
Shiny Red Tomatoes 173
short head of biceps femoris 160-161
shoulder
   common functional problems 52-54
   hip joint versus 151
   labral tears 49, 76, 99
   major structures 73-77
   nonthrowing stresses on 66
   throwing mechanics 65

shoulder muscles
   anterior treatments 93-95
   axiohumeral 86-88
   axioscapular 80-85
   posterior treatments 96-98
   scapulohumeral 88-93
skeletal muscle 9. *See also* muscles
skin rolling 39-40
sleep 210, 211
sliding filament theory 11-12
small hemipelvis 45
smooth muscle 9
soleus 191, 192-193, 194
somatic nervous system 24-25
sphincter muscles 10
spinal curvatures 44-45, 50-51
spinalis 136
spine
   common structural issues 44-45, 50-51
   muscles 115-121, 136-140
   structure 113-114, 133-134
spiraling
   abdomen 145, 146
   arm 105, 106
   technique described 38-39
   thigh 165, 168
splenius cervicis and capitis 120
split stance 34
squat position 34
stabilizers 10
sternoclavicular joint 74
sternocleidomastoid 127-128, 130-131
strain 5
strap muscles 10
stress, fascia response to 5-6
stress fractures 46, 196
stressors
   adductors 162, 163, 164
   anterior abdominal region 142-143, 144, 145
   anterior cervical muscles 128, 129
   axial skeleton 70

stressors (*continued*)
  axiohumeral muscles 86-88
  axioscapular muscles 81, 82, 83-85, 116-117
  elbow 98, 99, 100, 101-103, 104
  forearm 108, 109
  gluteal region 171, 172, 174, 175
  hamstrings 159-160, 161
  low back 137, 139-140
  lower extremity 67-70
  lower leg 186, 187, 188, 189, 190, 192, 193, 196, 197
  posterior cervical muscles 120, 121, 126
  quadriceps 156-157, 158
  scapulohumeral muscles 89-90, 91, 92, 93
  thigh 175, 176
  upper back and thorax 118-119
  upper extremity 64-67
structural problems
  common bone issues 44-46
  common joint issues 48-50
  common ligament issues 46-48
  manual therapy's role 43
  spinal 50-51
styloid process 130
suboccipital muscles 54, 125-126, 130, 132
suboccipital triangle 126
subscapularis 91, 97-98
subtalar joint 182
superficial cold applications 208-209
superficial fascia 31
superficial heat applications 209-210
superficial posterior compartment of lower leg 181, 191-195
superior nuchal line 130
supination of foot 69
supinator 103, 111
supraglenoid tubercle 99
supraspinatus 89-90, 96
Swedish massage 30, 34-38, 206

sympathetic nervous system 25-26, 27
syndesmosis sprain 183
synergists 9
synovial joints 73
synovial membrane of sternoclavicular joint 74
systemic contraindications 41

T
tactical athletes 63-64
talocrural joint 182
talus 182
tapotement 38
tarsal bones 183
tarsometatarsal joints 183
tender points 33
tendinopathy 53-54
tendinosis 59
tendinous inscriptions 158
tensegrity 5, 93
tensor fasciae latae 173, 175, 177-178
teres major 92, 97
teres minor 90-91
thenar eminence 109-110, 111
TheraCane 203
thermotherapy 209-210
thigh
  manual therapies 165-169, 176-179
  manual therapy cautions 166-167
  muscles 153, 155-164
thoracic outlet syndrome 85
thoracic spine structure 114
thoracolumbar aponeurosis 7, 87, 134-135
thoracolumbar fascia 7
throwing 64-66
thumb 79
tibia
  ACL actions on 47, 154
  connective tissue 7, 182
  deep posterior compartment 195
  joints 181, 182
  manual therapies 188, 198

manual therapy cautions 188
  menisci 48, 154
  pain along 59
  stress fractures 46
tibial artery, vein, and nerve 195, 198
tibialis anterior 185, 186
traction techniques
  abdomen 146-147, 148
  low back 141
  neck 132
  shoulder 93, 94
  thigh 166-167
transverse arch 183
transversospinalis muscle group 137-139
transversus abdominis 144-145, 147
trapezius 80-81, 115-116, 121-122
Trendelenburg gait 174
triceps brachii 102-103, 106
trigger points 23, 33, 213
trochlea of humerus 78
turf toe 187

U
ulnar collateral ligament tear 47-48
ulnar nerve 168
unipennate arrangements 10
upper back
  common causes of pain 53
  functional problems 54-55
  manual therapies 96-97, 121, 123, 132
  muscles 80-84, 115-119
upper cross syndrome 55
upper trapezius 80-81, 115, 116, 122, 124

V
varicose veins 213
vasoconstriction 27
vasodilation 27
vastus intermedius 157-158, 166
vastus lateralis 58, 154, 155, 156-157, 166
vastus medialis 58, 154, 155, 157, 166
venous system 18, 20
vertebrae 113-114, 133. *See also* spine
vertebral artery 126
vibrating foam rollers 207
vibration technique 38

W
whirlpools 210
whole-body cryotherapy 208
winging scapula 85
Wolff's law 60
wrist 78-79, 107-109

Z
z lines 12

About the Author

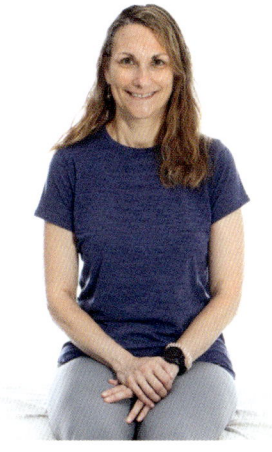

Portia B. Resnick, PhD, ATC, BCTMB, boasts 30 years of experience in the sports medicine field as a board-certified athletic trainer and massage therapist. With a PhD in education with a concentration in kinesiology from the University of Hawaii at Manoa, her research delved into the use of heart rate variability as a clinical measure of recovery in NCAA Division I athletes. Having worked as an athletic trainer at the high school, collegiate, and professional levels and as a sole proprietor in therapeutic and sports massage, she currently holds the positions of associate professor and coordinator of clinical education at California State University at Long Beach.

Dr. Resnick has held numerous volunteer and leadership positions in both the athletic training and massage communities. Her current research delves into sports massage, evidence-based practice in massage therapy, and massage ergonomics as part of her work for the Massage Therapy Foundation. She has given numerous presentations on manual therapy, the autonomic nervous system, and sports massage.

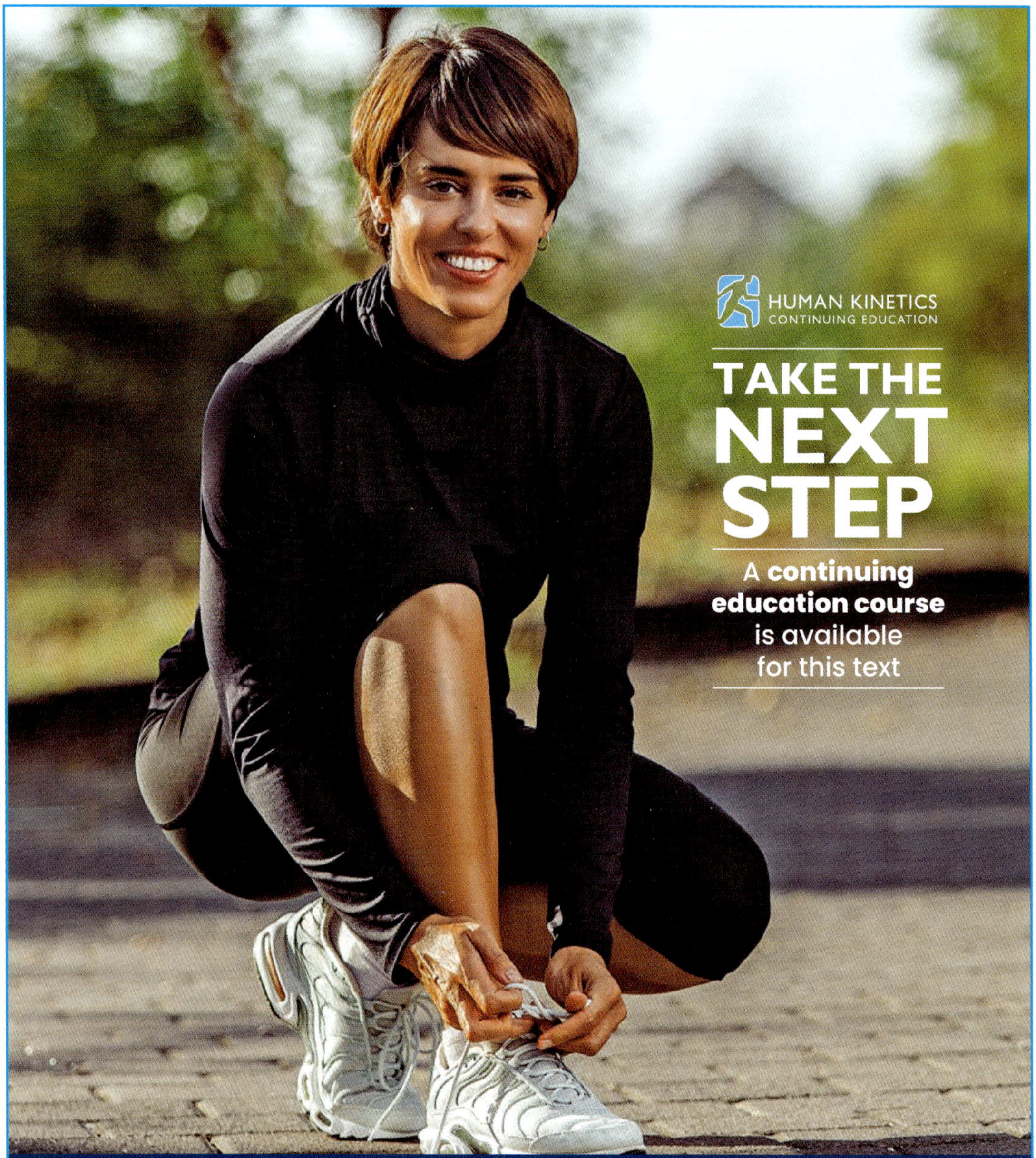

HUMAN KINETICS
CONTINUING EDUCATION

TAKE THE NEXT STEP

A **continuing education course** is available for this text

Find your CE course here:
US & International: US.HumanKinetics.com/collections/Continuing-Education
Canada: Canada.HumanKinetics.com/collections/Continuing-Education

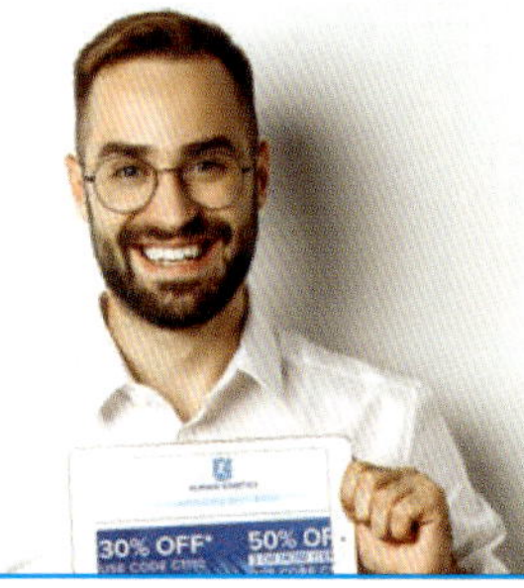

Subscribe to our newsletters today!

US

Canada

Get exclusive offers and stay apprised of CE opportunities.